Strategies for
Surviving Chemical Sensitivity:

the basics

by
Robert S. Mayer Ph.D.

Strategies for Surviving Chemical Sensitivities- the basics has been Printed on acid-free, recycled paper with soy-based ink.

This book offers suggestions for help in coping with:Chemical Sensitivity, Chemical Injury and Environmental Illness. The data, products, and suggestions in this book came from individuals who are chemically sensitive. The suggestions are "what worked" for them and are passed along in the hopes that these tips may be helpful for other individuals who have the same or similar problems.

Nothing in this book is to be taken as either medical or psychological advice by the author or publisher of this book. If medical of psychological services or treatment are needed, please seek the services of a competent professional provider.

ISBN: 978-0-578-05548-0

Printed in the United States of America by Graphic Solutions Group

To Randy:

Without whom all of this would not be possible

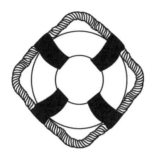

Contents

Introduction   ix

1. Basic Facts About Chemical Sensitivity   1

2. Finding a Physician   19

3. Treatment Options   41

4. Your Home   59

5. Your Bedroom   77

6. The Rest of the House   83

7. The Kitchen, Bathroom, Garage, and Utility Room   89

8. Personal Care Products   101

9. Finding a Safe Automobile   111

10. Managing Temporary Time Limited Exposures   119

11. To Move or Not to Move   129

12. To Build or Buy   147

13. Managing C.S. When Out of the House   159

14. Medical Problems   169

15. Having C.S. and Having Fun   185

Appendix   108

About the Author   200

About the Editor   202

About the Designer   204

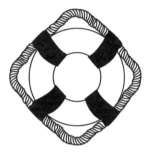

Introduction

The idea for this book is a product of the fertile brain of Cynthia Wilson, who is President of the Chemical Injury Information Network. A number of years ago, she ran a request in Our Toxic Times (OTT), the monthly publication of her organization, asking readers to send in information on products and ideas which helped them cope with their Chemical Sensitivity (CS). She then asked me to compile the results, which were subsequently published in a series of monthly articles in OTT. Each article, in addition to listing the products and ideas that the readership submitted, contained a request for additional products and ideas that were subsequently added to the original and comprise the central section of this work.

In another conversation with Mrs. Wilson she suggested that a simple, basic book about CS, explaining what it is, how it is diagnosed, the various treatments available, products that individuals have recommended, and psychological issues, was badly needed by the community, especially for newly diagnosed. *Strategies for Surviving Chemical Sensitivity* is the result of these two endeavors. That is what this book attempts to accomplish.

This book is not intended to be an encyclopedic recount of every aspect of this illness, nor a compete list of the multitude of resources and products for this patient population. It is a simple, get yourself started book, based upon reports sent in from individuals who claim to have found products and strategies that have helped them manage this illness. Readers who desire a fuller discussion of the medical, physical, psychological, legal, and political aspects of chemical poisoning are referred to *Multiple Chemical Sensitivity: A Survival Guide* by Pamela Reed Gibson, published by Earthrive Books, Churchville, Va., 2006. Individuals who are looking for a very complete list of products, suppliers, and web sites are referred to the encyclopedic work: *Less-Toxic Alternatives*, by Carolyn Gorman with Marie Hyde, published by Optimum Publishing, Hot Springs National Park, Arkansas, 2004. In addition, both of these works have excellent bibliographies for the reader who wishes to go still further.

As noted, the products suggested on the following pages, are those that certain individuals have found satisfactory. I also pass along the advice that I was given by Tad Taylor[1]. Tad was a unique man, who became a dear friend and mentor to me about this illness, and sadly, has recently passed away: "What works for one person, may not work for another. Test everything before you use or ingest it. Practice avoidance. And, conserve your resources."

Readers are also referred to *Our Toxic Times*, which publishes the latest theories and synopsis medical research concerning chemical sensitivity. The Chemical Information Injury Network, as quoted from their web site, CIIN.org, is a support and advocacy organization dealing with CS. It is run by the chemically injured for the benefit of the chemically injured, and focuses primarily on education, credible research into CS, and the empowerment of the chemically injured.

CIIN is a 501(C) non-profit, charitable, tax-exempt, membership organization; its resources are, with a few exceptions, reserved for its members. Becoming a member is simple - make a donation in any amount.

In addition, CIIN provides its members with:
• Expert Witness/Doctor referrals

• Attorney referrals

• A list of organization(s) in the state where the member resides

• A list of CIIN members for the state where the member resides

---

1. Justin Taylor has taken over his father's business and can be reached at www.healthy-homes.com.

- Referrals to experts in the fields of electromagnetic fields (EMFs), less-toxic pesticide and weed control, etc.
- CIIN's monthly newsletter, *Our Toxic Times*
- Materials for educational events, such as Earth Day booths
- Resource materials
- CIIN also has a very complete bibliography of medical literature and pamphlets, which can be obtained from them.

CIIN is also involved in:

- Educational support services for advancing the understanding of chemically related health problems, including MCS
- Providing testimony on state and federal legislation that directly impacts the MCS community and toxic concerns
- The Chemical Impact Project sponsored by the Tides Foundation
- Founding the National Coalition of the Chemical Injured
- Bringing national media attention to chemically-induced health issues
- Educating federal legislators on issues of concern to the MCS community
- Sponsoring national conferences on CS issues such as the development of MCS agenda priorities, a case definition for CS and other workshops.

To become a member of the Chemical Injury Information Network, go to their website's Membership Form page or call (406) 547-2255 to donate by MasterCard, Discover or Visa; or mail in a donation in any amount to CIIN, P.O. Box 301, White Sulphur Springs, MT 59645. (Suggested donations are: Fixed income - $15; Employed individuals - $30; Professionals - $50.) CIIN's activities are primarily supported by donations. An annual donation is necessary to maintain a membership and receive the newsletter.

I also wish to thank Cynthia and John Wilson for their support and encouragement, without which this book would not have been written. Also, to Treesha deFrance, my editor. In addition, much thanks is owed to my wife, Randy who also edited the text, created the cover design and laid out the book for printing. She also provided innumerable helpful suggestions along the way.

The resource information in this book was accurate at the time of writing but as with everything in this world, things change and product formulations change without notice.

Robert S. Mayer, Ph.D.
Monmouth Beach, N.J.
March 2010

Robert S. Mayer Ph.D.

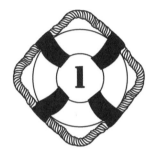

Basic Facts About Chemical Sensitivity
What is Chemical Sensitivity?

Chemical Sensitivity (CS) is a chronic, complicated, serious illness that is difficult to diagnose. It has many names. It is also known as Multiple Chemical Sensitivity (MCS), Chemical Injury (CI), Environmental Illness (EI), Toxicant Induced Loss of Tolerance (TILT), Toxic Injury (TI), and Idiopathic Environmental Intolerance (EIT). At present, there is no cure for Chemical Sensitivity. However, with proper diagnosis and management, one can have a relatively symptom free, productive life.

The numerous names for this condition illustrate the failure of the medical professionals to come to an agreement on the basics of this illness. At this writing there is little agreement on a case definition, causes, natural history, prognosis and treatment of Chemical Sensitivity. Consequently this serious condition is not well accepted, nor is it understood by many members of the medical community and general public. The negative consequences to afflicted individuals seeking treatment and validation might be misdiagnosis, leading to improper treatment, which at best would do nothing for the individual seeking help, and at worst, lead to increased physical and emotional suffering.

The names, "Chemical Sensitivity" and "Multiple Chemical Sensitivity" most accurately describe the condition since they include the word "chemical." People with Chemical Sensitivity (PWCS) experience physical and psychological symptoms resulting from exposure to various chemical substances.

Symptoms and Progress of the Illness

The physical symptoms caused by a chemical exposure generally include one or more of the following: headache, brain fog, fatigue, muscle aches, food intolerances, and/or breathing difficulties. In essence, in a chemically sensitive individual, chemical exposure to chemicals can affect any system in the body. This includes: the neurological, gastrointestinal, endocrine, musculoskeletal, immunological, urological, cardiovascular, metabolic, psychological, and reproductive systems.

Over time many PWCS may become increasingly sensitive and symptomatic when exposed to very low concentrations of a symptom producing substance. For PWCS, the concentration of the toxin required to trigger a reaction is well below those that can be detected by a non Chemically Sensitive person. They are also well below levels deemed safe by the medical community, chemical industry, and state and federal agencies. The symptom causing substances most commonly cited by PWCS are volatile organic compounds (VOCs) which are found in: petrochemicals, plastics, automobile exhaust, pesticides, paints, solvents, building materials, and many other products.

Unfortunately, other types of symptom producing substances are found in many commonly used commercial household and personal products, such as: detergents, deodorants, hair coloring, fragrances, fabric softeners, synthetic and treated fabrics. Since petrochemical by-products are extensively used in an industrial society, the list of possible offenders is extensive, and grows every year.

A PWCS can be sensitive to a few substances or to a variety of related or chemically unrelated ones. This later individual is often inaccurately termed a universal reactor. A better term, although not as commonly used, is a "highly reactive individual." [1]

Depending on the nature of the chemical and the damage it created, CS may be contained or progressive. It can be anything from annoying to debilitating. Reports of this problem parallel the increasing prevalence of chemicals in our chemically polluted, society.

---

1. It is improbable, if not impossible to react to everything.

Characteristics of the Illness

Chemical Sensitivity manifests itself differently in different individuals. In some PWCS, the physical reactions are limited to one or a few substances such as perfume or tobacco smoke. Many seemingly unrelated substances affect others. In addition, as the illness progresses, very often, very small concentrations of the offending substance cause symptoms. Since nerves are central to all bodily systems, their sensitization might cause the "spreading" phenomenon that has been reported by sufferers and demonstrated in animal research. Because of this, some PWCS become highly sensitive. They react to almost everything they come into continued contact with.

A physical reaction to an offending substance can be immediate, or delayed. An immediate reaction after exposure to a substance allows one to easily determine what made one sick, and thus what to avoid.

Delayed reactions occur a period of time after the exposure, making it more difficult to isolate the cause of the symptom. Without a simple cause and effect relationship, a delayed reaction can feed either the "I must be crazy" theory or "There is a yet to be detected physical problem wrong with me." Careful detailed diary keeping, listing exposures and symptoms, over a long enough period of time can often tease out the culprit.

Many PWCS report a heightening of some or all of their senses. The heightening of the senses might be either a warning mechanism to alert the individual of danger, or a by product of the illness. As the individual understands that chemicals are making them sick, they will gradually remove noxious toxic items from their environment. As a result, their sense of smell is exposed to fewer strong and harmful odors. They become more sensitive or better able to distinguish what causes their symptoms. This phenomenon is called "unmasking". When the smell organs receive many scents at the same time, they tend to either counteract each other or dull ("mask"). PWCS call this phenomenon "masking". Perfume salespeople understand this. They are taught never to put more than three different scents on an individual or they will lose the sale as the customer's sense of smell gets "masked" and their mind confused. An individual who goes on a sugar free diet for a while and then eats a sugary substance will notice that at first it does not taste good and milder sweets, such as natural fruit are indeed very sweet. Obviously, if you are diabetic, whether the sugar tastes sweet, good, or bad, it is still harmful to your medical condition. For the PWCS, masking might lead to a failure to recognize that their detoxification and neurological systems are being damaged.

An example is being in a room, with many people talking at the same time. Individual words may not be understandable, but the ear *is* being assaulted. If the volume is loud enough, such as at a rock concert, audible damage may occur. If the injured individual recognizes the cause of their symptoms and removes themselves from the source, at some point, the reaction will abate.

A person's recovery time is dependent on the magnitude and duration of the exposure, the amount of damage that has been done to the system as well as the genetic/biological/psychological status of the body. Recovery time is the amount of time it takes from getting sick from an exposure to feeling better. In many individuals, avoidance of "chemical insults" for a "long enough" period of time stabilizes them. This can allow what is rebuildable to rebuild, or at the very least, further damage is arrested.

As this happens, the person gradually improves so that they can tolerate more and more exposures. In this healthier state, their recovery time shortens, and they are to tolerate more things and live a more "normal life."

The amount of improvement is individual. It depends on: the genetic/biological/psychological status of the body; the particular nature of the chemical that injured them; and how long they remained in a "toxic" situation before they adopted a life style with as much avoidance of toxic chemical exposure as possible.

In this way, many chemically injured people have been able to create a safe living place, find ways to manage their illnesses, and get on with their lives, although most often their new life is a different one than they once imagined it would be.

For others the course is more difficult. For many it is very difficult to obtain an environmentally "safe" or even tolerable place in which to live and work. Many do not have enough money to live on. To compound their misery, their co-workers, friends and family might not understand the nature of the illness or not believe them. The medical profession, which, by definition exists to help them, is as unknowledgeable in recognizing this illness, as they are untrained in treating it. Because of this physicians attempting to treat what they do not understand, often violate their own cardinal medical rule of "Do no harm." Without the basic survival needs being met, the PWCS's life becomes a constant desperate, sometimes frantic, struggle to find air to breath, a car to drive, food to eat, water to drink, and employment to get enough money to live on.

Charlatans and quacks sprout in abundance in the fertile field of a chronic, debilitating illness without a specific cure. Unfortunately, more often than not, they relieve the sufferer of their money rather than their symptoms.

As in all illnesses a small percentage, around 2%, spontaneously recover. Some PWCS report having been "cured" by God or a spiritual healer, as the discarded wheel chairs and crutches lining the approaches to various healing shrines around the world attest. Yet for most, a spiritual cure does not occur, or God has chosen not to intervene. God's absence adds additional fertilizer to the already fertile field in which unethical faith healers profitably till.

Theories About the Causes of Chemical Sensitivity

It is obvious that exposure to certain chemicals cause various physical and psychological symptoms in many people. Well known examples are: tobacco, ether, carbon tetrachloride, dry cleaning solvent, formaldehyde, paints, alcohol, carbon monoxide, carbon dioxide, pesticides, recreational drugs, and anti-personnel gases. All of the above can get people sick. If the dose is high enough, they can cause permanent disability or death.

Therefore, the statement that chemicals are harmful, as well as beneficial cannot be in dispute. The dispute focuses on the causation and mechanism of CS. What is it in certain people that make them react to chemicals in concentrations so minute to be undetectable by general public? Why are some permanently damaged, and others just mildly ill or uncomfortable? And why do many people who use these products all the time never get ill?

These contradictory, confusing observations have led many individuals, the sick and non-sick, to question the validity of CS. The non-CS person often questions the motivation and mental health of a PWCS who says that chemicals, including such common items as deodorants or perfumes, make them sick.

The non-CS deodorant wearer, when confronted, generally says something like: "Since you are telling me that you get sick from the same product that I use all the time, and asking me not to use it in your presence, you must either be trying to manipulate me or you are crazy." Many get angry, interpreting a comment about their scented product such as "You stink", as a personal affront.

Given the nature of the human being, this is a reasonable, although illogical response. In the history of all illnesses, even lethal ones such as the Black Death or the influenza pandemic of the 1920's which killed twice as many people as the First World War, some individuals have been more affected than others. Many were not bothered even as they cared for the ill. If this were not true, I would not be here to write this book, nor you to read it.

Many scientists accept the reality of CS and have been, in spite of a scarcity of funds, investigating its causes, mechanisms, and possible treatment modalities. At this stage of the process, they are not in agreement and there are several theories proposed and under exploration. These theories include:

Damage to the Enzymatic Detoxification System: Lately, researchers have been focusing on the way in which the human system detoxifies potentially harmful substances. Toxic substances constantly enter the body through the nose, lungs, skin, and alimentary canal. To combat this, the human body has an intricate, complex, enzymatic system. This system, when working properly, converts these potentially harmful substances to inert ones that can be eliminated by the body's normal pathways. This school of thought believes that a person living in the chemical soup that comprises today's world did not develop the human detoxification system for use. Thus, a system that has been genetically weakened or toxically insulted gets overloaded, damaged, and can even break.

When this happens, the toxic substances break through the blood/brain barrier, or enter the brain directly through the nose. Given the nature of the chemical or its concentration, the toxin can act as destructively on brain cells as a loose cannon acts on an 18th Century warship. Resultant brain damage can be demonstrated through SPECT (Single Photon Emission Computed Tomography) and PET (Positron Emission Tomography) scans of the afflicted individual's brain, as well as QEEG (Qualitative Electroencephalogram). In PWCS, these tests demonstrate damage to various parts of the brain, and/or restricted blood flow. This phenomenon is usually prevalent in the frontal lobes.

Further credence is given to this theory is the use of it by some of the pesticide and biological warfare manufacturers. The biochemists employed by those firms study the enzymatic system of the organism they want to kill, and develop chemicals that will defeat the system. They also note that the certain chemicals injure or destroy human beings. Chemicals have been used in warfare far back in antiquity. Everyone knows that Paris killed Achilles in his one vulnerable spot, his heel, with a poisoned arrow during the Siege of Troy.

Neural Sensitization: Dr. Iris Bell proposed that CS may be the result of nerve sensitization. Sensitization is an enhancement of neurochemical responses to stimulants. It is seen in rats and can be induced in humans by the repeated use of various substances. In CS, neurological pathways may be sensitized, and therefore hypersensitive to stimulation, since chemicals can cause chronic damage to body biochemistry. This theory converges with the Elevated Nitric Oxide/Peroxynitrite Vicious Cycle Paradigm of Dr. Martin Pall, Washington State University, explains how certain chemical exposures can initiate a sequence that can lead to neural sensitization. The chemicals in question are: organophosphate/carbamate pesticides, volatile organic solvents, pyrethroid pesticides and organochlorine pesticides, all of which are reported to produce CS and trigger symptoms in PWCS.

Neurogenic Inflammation: Dr. William Meggs relates the process of neurogenic inflammation to CS. Inflammation is a biological process initiated by many things, allergens, infection, and injury. Typically, inflammation causes tissue alteration. Neurogenic inflammation is a subset of inflammation, initiated by stimulation of c-fiber nerves, which release neuropeptides. Signs of inflammation then occur at sites other than the site of the original stimulus, including central processes, parasympathetic and sympathetic reflexes. This theory applies to CS in that the chemosensitive nerves, their products, and their receptors are altered, and that the alterations account for the increased sensitivity seen in CS. One study showed PWCS had an augmented inflammatory response to chemical exposure.

Immune System Dysfunction: This is an older theory that is not accepted by the current, up to date group of researchers and practitioners. The immune system obviously allows an individual to cure, or resist illness. Deficient immune systems can even attack the body causing autoimmune illnesses. The immunological theory assumes that an individual contracts CS due to a deficient immune system. The immune deficiency is thought to be due to genetics, poor nutrition, or that it has broken down after an assault or overload by some external substance. When that happens, the immune system generates an immune response which can affect other organs of the body. The individual who sneezes and gets a runny nose upon contact with an allergen is a simple, well-recognized example of an immune response. While this is a logical theory as the immune system controls illness, a definable acceptable marker has yet to be found.

The Allergic Theory: Building on the immune theory, some researchers and clinicians view the illness as a "brain allergy", and write books with catchy titles such as *Allergic to the 21st Century*. Practitioners who hold this theory often tend to be allergists or immunologists, and treat the condition within their medical specialty model. Sadly, by attempting to treat it within an allergic paradigm, they might very well make the PWCS worse.

In practice, the immune system camp, tries to correct the immune deficiency by various methods. Some use so called immune boosters. Others try and reduce the total load on the immune system by desensitizing the individual to known allergens. Another group use homeopathic anti-allergic techniques, in which it is thought that minute doses of the offending substance will stop the reaction, a sort of "hair of the dog that bit me" theory. This later procedure is called Provocative Neutralization and will be discussed in greater detail in the "treatment" section of this work.

As of this writing, although many practitioners use these techniques, the results have not proven successful in enough cases to justify the cost. In some cases the chemicals used to build up the immune system, or antigens used to desensitize an individual to a supposed allergen or a known toxic chemical have even been harmful. This might be because most PWCS tend to get sensitive to anything they are in continual exposure to, including the herbs used to build the immune system, antigen tests, or desensitization injections. The later is reported to have a greater high harm to help ratio if they are preserved in chemicals, such a phenol and glycerin, than those that are preservative free.[2] Furthermore, after exhaustive study of the immune systems of chemically sensitive individuals and those who are not, enough evidence has not been found to draw any scientifically valid or useable conclusions.

Chemical or Nutritional Imbalance: This theory assumes that there are various substances such as vitamins, minerals, enzymes, fatty acids, and micronutrients that are missing in the affected individual's bio system. These ingredients are necessary for the proper functioning of the entire system, especially the detoxification system. Thus if any are missing or deficient, illness, in this case CS, occurs.

The popularity of this theory for this illness as well as others is attested

---

2. See Gibson synopsis of "Survey of Perceived Treatment Efficacy for Conventional and Alternative Therapies Reported by Persons with Chemical Sensitivity" in the appendix.

to by the enormous supplement and health food industry, and the sufferer's endless search for a "magic pill." Yet after extensive and expensive tests of PWCS for any missing nutrients, and after the addition of the supposed missing ingredients into their diet, there are not enough positive results to prove the theory.

Genetic Predisposition: This theory holds more promise although it was discovered under tragic circumstances. Many soldiers who fought in the Gulf War in 1991 started to complain of CS-like symptoms. Even though an obvious cause and effect exists between the toxicity of the war zone ablaze in oil fires, and reported illness, the Federal Government and American military denied for years that there was such a thing as Gulf War Syndrome. They preferred to label it Post Traumatic Stress Disorder, which took the cause out of the physical and moved it to the psychological. This gave the government an excuse to refuse to research the condition or treat the victims.

Eventually the government did come around and appropriated funds to research the condition. Unfortunately it took over ten years of extensive pressure from sick veterans, the very same individuals who put their lives on the line for their country. Once on board, the federal government embarked upon a treatment and research program to prove the validity of the soldier's complaints. During the research, they found a genetic difference between the chemically sensitive and non-chemically sensitive soldiers. However, even though it is logical to suppose that the afflicted veterans had a genetic predisposition, researchers have not been able to compare the genetic structure of the same individual before and after chemical exposure. In addition studies have shown that exposure to various organic chemicals can create over 100 changes in genetic expression—thirty-five of which can become permanent.

The unanswered question is "Are some people more apt to contract the condition due to a genetic abnormality or did the chemicals cause the genetic difference?" At the moment, the best that can be said is that there certainly could be a genetic predisposition to become sensitive to chemicals, as well as that chemicals can affect genetic changes.

All this may be a moot point. The genetic theory, even if true, does not lead to a treatment/prevention protocol, except genetic testing to give prospective parents the choice of whether to gamble inflicting this illness on their future offspring.

Porphyria: Inherited or Acquired Porphyria is a deficiency in the enzyme system that is responsible for supplying the proper amount of oxygen to the tissues. Porphyria can be either genetic, or caused by drugs, chemicals, infections, or malnutrition. Dr. Gordon Baker of Seattle, Washington found that about half of his chemically sensitive patients tested positively for Porphyria. At present, while Porphyria is a medically accepted condition, there is no known medical treatment or cure.

Long Term Use of Antibiotics and Steroids: This theory argues that excessive use of these products alters the bacterial flora of the intestinal tract and causes an overgrowth of yeast, specifically Candida Albicans. The yeasts, as they go about their lives in the body, emit toxins and disrupt the normal bacterial balance in the intestinal tract. The resulting condition, called Candidiasis, can interfere with absorption of nutrients from food. In addition, these toxins can also damage the stomach lining. Some clinicians think that a damaged intestinal lining allows undigested, undetoxified food molecules to pass directly into the blood system. They term this condition "Leaky Gut." This theory, unproven, and disputed by many, it is thought by the believers to be responsible for the high incidence of food sensitivities reported by the chemically injured population.

Candidiasis, an overgrowth of yeast in the intestinal canal, is a well-known and accepted medical condition. There are drugs on the market to treat it, along with an accepted dietary protocol. However, although many PWCS also have Candidiasis, successful treatment of the latter, does not cure the former. Current researchers believe that Candidiasis is a result of CS--not the cause.

Undiagnosed Lyme Disease: Lyme Disease can masquerade as other illnesses which obviously further confuses this already confused issue. The professionals who hold this theory argue that the increase in PWCS has paralleled the increase in the number of cases of Lyme Disease. They conclude that CS is really Lyme Disease in disguise. To compound maters, Lyme Disease is very difficult to diagnose and often resistant to treatment. In spite of this, some clinicians, in the absence of conclusive proof, treat an CS patient as if they have Lyme Disease, rather than CS. To treat the Lyme Disease, they prescribe a long term course of antibiotics.

Sometimes curing the suspected Lyme Disease also cures the patient of their CS. More often it does not. The long term use of antibiotics necessary to treat Lyme Disease can further sensitize the PWCS and lead to an exacerbation of symptom, by causing Candidiasis, in an already chemically sensitive individual.

Eastern Medicine: Others, either by predilection or out of frustration with Western medicine, take an Eastern approach. Using ancient Chinese medicine as a base, they believe there is a disturbance or blockage in the vital life energy flow, called Chi, of the sufferer. They then employ practices designed to unblock this energy such as acupuncture, various ritualized movements and Chinese herbs. A glance at the result of various treatment surveys included in this book will show that this approach goes no further to proving the cause than previously mentioned ones. In addition there is the possibility of sensitivity reactions to the various herbs.

Parasites: The possibility of an organism living rent free in your body is a wild card which could be a reality. Parasites can do all sorts of damage to an infected individual's system. Unfortunately tests to detect parasites, which are not all that accurate, are not routinely performed during a physical examination nor has enough research on this possibility been done.[3]

Psychological Theories: A minority, but vocal body of researchers and writers with access to the microphone, shout that CS is a psychological illness. They argue that psychological problems either predispose an individual to chemical sensitivity, or the complainers are using the excuse of being chemically sensitive, consciously or unconsciously, to obtain a secondary gain. Common secondary psychological gains are sympathy, special treatment, being taken care of, being special, or having a reason to exist, to mention an obvious few.

While no one can deny the interplay between the psychological and physical, there is scant evidence to indicate that the former caused the later. In fact, studies show that psychotherapy has not been effective in treating this illness. For a large number of PWCS, being labeled and treated psychologically, especially with psychotropic drugs, has been harmful.[4] The harm can come from psychotropic drugs, which are chemicals most PWCS react to, or unproven behavior modification therapy in which PWCS are told that they should expose themselves

---

3. Some parasites can be diagnosed by blood tests; others have to be "caught" in stool samples.

4. According to the Gibson survey, the use of psychotropic drugs to treat CS is listed among the most harmful of the reported treatments with a help harm ratio of. Psychotherapy fares little better.

to chemicals to "break" the fear pattern, or to "build up tolerance". It would be more therapeutic for the psychological profession to focus their attention on assisting PWCS with the psychological effects of this illness, rather than hypothesizing a psychological cause, and proceeding along a potentially harmful treatment protocol. Interestingly, the medical communities of Austria and Germany have defined CS as physical not psychological.

Conclusion: Therefore, the current most logical causative theory of Chemical Sensitivity is a chemical insult to the susceptible individual's enzymatic detoxification system. When this happens the individual is no longer protected against further toxic assaults. Toxic chemicals break through the blood brain barrier, or enter directly through the nasal cavity, damage the central nervous system, and cause physical symptoms. This is a theory of disease that a researcher Dr. Claudia Miller at the University of Texas named: Toxic Induced Loss of Tolerance, or TILT.

Other Related Conditions

A percentage of PWCS become sensitive to electromagnetic fields (EMFs), a very difficult problem to manage in our electronic world. These fields are all around us in the form of electricity in our homes and vehicles. EMFs are present around electrical wiring, appliances, high tension wires, and microwave transmissions from innumerable, ever increasing wireless devices such as radios, cell phones, satellites, and computers.

It is obvious that EMFs are all pervasive in our society. They comprise a dimension that we cannot see, however it is a dimension which some people feel. This fourth dimension is an invisible, potentially harmful web of electrical and radio waves, most prevalent in built-up industrial urban areas, but increasingly crisscrossing the country, and eventually the globe. Very little research has been done on the long-term effects of these fields, or what constitutes a safe level, yet many individuals can attest to the ill health effects from them.

Trying to live in a world that consists of a chemical and electrical stew is difficult for the chemically and/or electromagnetically sensitive individual. Most PWCS have difficulty finding a "safe" place (defined by the CS community as a chemical or EMF-free environment) in which to live, work, and even breathe. Unfortunately, chemicals and EMFs are here to stay and PWCS hoping their use will decline is about as realistic as expecting to live long enough for evolution to adapt their bodies to be resistant to them.

There also seems to be a not yet fully understood overlap between CS and other illnesses that have similar symptoms such as: Fibromyalgia, Multiple Chemical Sensitivity, Chronic Fatigue Syndrome, Gulf War Syndrome, World Trade Center Syndrome and Sick Building Syndrome. Even though similar enzymatic detoxification deficiencies have been found in all five conditions, arguments abound whether the above conditions are: all different manifestations of the same illness with the same causative mechanisms; similar but different illnesses; or physical or psychological conditions. At some point the various hypothesis will be proven or disproved by the scientific method, and the truth will be known.

Demographics of CS
Studies show that this condition is present in all societies that use chemicals, which is most of the world. It is estimated that up to one third of the population are afflicted to one degree or another.[5] In the so called third world, where chemicals may or may not be used in as large quantities as the industrial world, statistical reporting technology is not developed to a degree where the prevalence can be known.

Not surprisingly, the illness is more prevalent in individuals who work in closed, non-ventilated places which contain toxic fumes, or factories that process harsh chemicals. Examples of such workplaces are hospitals, schools, oil refineries, and plastic factories to mention an obvious few.

Others speculate that there is a genetic component, as the condition seems to run in families or individuals that are biologically related. This phenomenon, although reported, has not yet been scientifically validated.

There is no significant age, ethnic or racial differences in this illness. No accurate head count has been done on the number of men who are chemically sensitive verses the number of women. However, it is believed that women are more susceptible than men. This may be because the available studies have been done predominantly on women, or it may be that more women develop CS.

If there are indeed a disproportionate percentage of females, it may be due to the fact that men have more of the enzymes necessary for detoxification than women. Men also have less internal estrogens, and a woman's enzymatic detoxification system (the Redox system) is frailer than a child's, therefore, it might be easier to poison a woman than a man.

---

5. Meggs, W.J., Dunn, K.A., Bloch R.M., Goodman, P.E., Davidoff, A.L.: "Prevalence and Nature of Allergy and Chemical Sensitivity in a General Population." *Archives of Environmental Health*, 1996, Jul-Aug; 51(4):275-282.

Other Hypotheses for the Disproportionate Number of Women with the Illness Include:

The body fat theory: Women have more body fat than men, so women tend to store unprocessed, oil-soluble chemicals. These chemicals are released into the blood stream slowly, and get the woman sick.

The cowboy's are tough theory: It is more accepted in Western society for women to talk about feelings and illnesses than men. Men are trained to be "tough." Therefore, a woman is more prone to discuss her problem than is a man who will try and "be a man" and "tough it out", and not admit "weakness".

The women are exposed to more chemicals than men theory: Many women are exposed to more household cleaners, detergents, fabric softeners, and cosmetics than men. Even though it is changing, women in the work force are still more likely to be working in the room containing the copier, printer, and fax machine, a room loaded with toxic fumes. They also tend to be in closer, confined contact with other women who are using cosmetics and other chemical products which they inhale.

The sweat theory: Men, more so than women, tend to engage in hard physical outdoor labor. By breathing fresh air and sweating, they have a better chance of processing the chemicals while they work. This prevents them from building up in the body and harming it. Obviously, this theory assumes that while working, they process more toxins than they retain.

Reactions of the General Public and the Medical Profession

People with CS are sensitive to common products that most people are not sensitive to. Because these products impact their health, attempts to avoid them limit their lives in innumerable ways. This sensitivity is a phenomenon outside the experience of the non-afflicted.

Since the non-afflicted includes most members of the helping professions, family and friends, it is very difficult for the PWCS to obtain proper treatment, understanding, and support from relatives and friends. This often results in greater physical and psychological suffering for the already suffering PWCS. Worse yet is the probability of being misdiagnosed and mistreated. Improper diagnosis and treatment can cause the illness to progress. In some cases, this leads to total disability, which might have been avoided with proper care.

This lack of the traditional medical and scientific communities' agreement as to the cause, in fact as to physical reality of the illness, has resulted in the illness being misunderstood, and denied. This may be a normal situation common for all relatively newly discovered illnesses. All new illnesses go through a transitional period during which they are questioned, denied, seen as a spiritual failure, or judged as psychological. At some point an undeniable relationship between cause and illness is proven and the "new" medical condition legitimized. Once legitimized, it is added to the official diagnostic lists, assigned an official number, included in medical school curricula, and added to required continuing education courses. In this slow, but normal, process the medical community is educated and the sufferer has a better chance of obtaining proper diagnosis and treatment. As the information eventually filters down to the general public, the sufferers will have a better chance to obtain support, understanding, and the "crazy" label will be dropped.

Examples of the above process in previously not commonly accepted medical conditions are well known. A few that deserve brief mention are: the tobacco/cancer relationship, the germ theory of disease, Black Lung disease, Multiple Sclerosis, and Hysteria.

The relationship between tobacco and cancer has been known since 1924. Denial of this relationship by the tobacco industry, medical community and general public, reinforced by voluminous industry financed "scientific" studies, and "doctor testimonials", caused many needless deaths. The denial was so strong that the even the numerous cancer related deaths of the tobacco-using owners of the major tobacco companies, the Marlboro Man, and Lucky Strike Girl, failed to break it.

Years ago people could not comprehend that disease, infections, and even death were caused by unclean, unsanitary conditions. Many people believed that bathing more than twice a year was dangerous to an individual's health. Rather than wash with soap and water, they sprayed perfume. One can only wonder how many people died while vehemently arguing that bathing or cleaning a wound was bad for their health. During the American Civil War, the great majority of individuals who were wounded died from infections caused by unsanitary operating conditions. The American Civil War surgeon would remove his knife from between his teeth where he was holding it, proceed to cut off another limb from his next patient, wipe the bloody knife on his soiled apron, and put it back between his teeth, as he prepared for the next amputation. Eventually, the role of germs in disease transmission was uncovered and lives saved.

Black Lung Disease, now known to be caused by coal dust, was missed for over 125 years because it didn't show up on an X-ray. Multiple Sclerosis (MS) was called Hysterical Paralysis for over 100 years, and now it's also been proven that in some cases, MS is caused by solvent exposure.

Hysteria, which is an older term for a variety of different psycho/physical conditions, has gone through many transitions. The Ancient Greeks thought that the condition was restricted to women and caused by a wandering uterus. Yes, you read that right. Unknowledgeable about human anatomy, they simply assumed that the afflicted woman's uterus had "wandered" for one reason or another, to another place in her body. To cure the condition they reasoned that the uterus had to be induced to travel back to where it belonged. To facilitate this process, they applied noxious substances to the suspected new uterine residence. If this didn't work, they applied pleasant smelling things to the vagina in an attempt to induce the uterus to return to where it belonged.

The Victorians, following their sexist predecessors, also thought Hysteria was restricted to women, but with a better knowledge of female anatomy, believed it was caused by childhood sexual abuse. Others believed it was because the women were sexually deprived, or repressed. The cure to them, was obvious. The psychiatric profession now sees Hysteria as group of non-gender specific, psychological illnesses that can have physical as well as emotional causes or symptoms.

Sadly, societies are slow to change their ways. In the Middle Ages, it wasn't until sewage flowed from the streets over the door sills and into the houses that the towns allocated money and energy to construct adequate waste removal systems. And everyone knows that George Washington was bled in an attempt to cure his throat infection. At that time bleeding as a treatment was medically accepted, and widely used -- George Washington died.

In the case of CS, an additional factor for the lack of recognition and resulting acceptance of the illness might be an attempt to protect what appears to be the cause of the problem-chemicals. Our society's industrial, economic and cultural systems are built and based on chemicals. To accept the fact that the very chemicals, which have made this nation and other industrial nations profitable and powerful are harmful to our health, is economically and psychologically threatening for most people. They believe that chemicals are obviously not harmful to them, as they observe that they, and the rest of the society, do not react to those "so called toxic products." The naysayer's obvious conclusion is, that the CS individual, who says that they react to something that the non-CS individual uses without having a reaction, lies someplace on the continuum between threatening and crazy.

Afflicted individuals are in a difficult transitional state by the lack of medical, scientific and societal acceptance of the dangers of chemicals. This reduces their options for help and support. Fortunately, enough is now known and accepted by a portion of the professional community so that methods are available for treatment, education, and support. There is also an extensive on-line educational network, organizations, newsletters, and local support groups for PWCS. This has enabled the knowledgeable to arrest the negative progression of the illness and find ways to manage the condition and achieve a life of fulfillment within a life of avoidance.

Robert S. Mayer Ph.D.

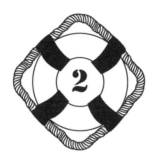

Finding a Physician

The Problem:

Physicians that specialize in Chemical Sensitivity are in short supply and can be counted on the fingers of one hand. To compound the problem these specialists are scattered throughout the United States and difficult to locate. Given the small number of specialists, these doctors are most likely located outside of the patient's immediate or comfortable travel zone. This geographic reality presents the PWCS, struggling to find clean air in which to breathe and live, with the additional problems of safe travel, and safe housing along the way. Also, if one has to stay near the doctor, to undergo evaluation, testing or treatment, finding tolerable, (nontoxic) accommodations are essential but limited.[1]

There are board certified licensed physicians, practicing mainstream medicine, that are familiar with Chemical Sensitivity. Unfortunately, they represent the minority of the medical profession and their declared specialty, or subspecialty in CS, is not listed in the little black book that your family physician uses to find referrals.

---

1. Air travel can also be problematical as the air in the confined space of an airplane is typically bad. One might be seated next to an individual wearing fragrance, and arriving at one's destination find that the car rental agency only has automobiles that have been cleaned with toxic chemicals.

Easier to locate, usually found, unfortunately after a series of fruitless, frustrating, consultations with members of the above, or what this book will term "the official community" are physicians that practice "alternative medicine." This group, for whatever reasons, seems to be more familiar, and accepting of this condition than members of the official community.

Alternative medicine practitioners include: Some conventional medical practitioners; members of the American Academy of Environmental Medicine; Chiropractors; Naturopaths; Homeopaths; Faith Healers; Herbalists; acupuncturists and other groups. Some of their treatments and medical interventions are not recognized, nor qualify for reimbursement by an insurance company and generally not respected by the official medical community.[2]

Thus, while many of the alternative practitioners are willing to look at things "out of the box", their diagnosis does not carry the same weight as a member of the American Medical Association, the American Academy of Allergy and Immunology, or other such gold standard organizations both of which, at this writing do not, recognize CS as a legitimate illness.[3] Therefore, most practicing physicians are unfamiliar with CS as a legitimate illness, unable to recognize it, unable to accept it, and unable to treat it. Those that heroically try, often make their patient worse.

Before one starts to wander down the non productive path of anger which can increase your symptoms, the reality is that any newly reported illness gets incorporated slowly in the medical profession. This is done in order to protect the public health from charlatans. Ironically, such time delays result in lack of proper diagnosis and treatment, which often results in damage to patients seeking treatment, and to public health.

On a hopeful note, progress is slowly being made. After six years of official denial, the city of New York set up three diagnostic centers for victims of the 2001 World Trade Center disaster. Perhaps the combined pressure of the Gulf War veterans, and a disaster that was visible on TV, at home, and affected people one knew, rather than some far away place, sped things up. The image of the toxic cloud hovering above the fallen towers was as pungent to the eyes and psyches of the TV viewers as the air was to anyone living in or downwind of New York City. This was not an event that happened to a "volunteer" army in some far away place that many people needed a map to locate.

---

2. See the help/harm ratio in the survey of various treatments found in the appendix.

3. One wonders if the doubting members of the medical community have read a newspaper after the Gulf war of 1991 or even are aware of the illnesses following the events of September 11, 2001.

The main reason that there are so few knowledgeable physicians to diagnose and treat this illness is because CS is not included in the standard medical school curriculum. It is not there because CS is not an officially recognized affliction with a scientifically proven cause, prognosis, and treatment. For example, the American Medical Association and the American Academy of Allergy and Immunology do not recognize it. The reasoning of these organizations is that, although it might exist, CS might be a psychological problem, or an urban myth. They rest their decision on the fact that even though there are patient and physician reports, not enough double blind studies, the medical scientific gold standard, have been done to allow them to bestow their official seal of approval on this diagnosis.[4]

The physicians treating the illness would have to agree that there is a scarcity of peer-reviewed documentation. However, they defend the meager scientific research by saying that they are too busy with the deluge of patients needing treatment to spend their time doing research. In addition, research is expensive and few organizations have come forward with money. Most of the financing for medical research comes from the pharmaceutical industry or the government, neither, of which have the motivation or interest to prove that profitable and essential chemicals are causing a public health epidemic. Thus, for obvious reasons, they have not been anxious to investigate this illness, and prefer it to be a psychological one for which a psychotropic drug can be prescribed.

It is a sad fact that after seventeen years of reports by physicians and complaints by injured veterans, the federal government is just starting to research Gulf War Syndrome. The lengthy government denial of veteran's illnesses from reports of Agent Orange poisoning from the 1963-1973 war in Viet Nam is another terrible example of federal agencies unethically protecting themselves at the expense of the citizenry, in this case soldiers that risked their lives in service to their country.

Even though every PWCS knows that chemicals make them sick and avoidance of chemicals make them feel better, the official medical community and population at large have been slow to accept this fact. As noted in Chapter I, this lack of acceptance has been true with virtually all new illnesses. At first they are denied, and refused admittance into the

---

4. Progress might be occurring as, the most prestigious of these groups, the American Medical Association is currently on the fence regarding this illness. It has retracted its initial rejection and is now taking a "We need more research" approach.

hallowed chambers of "legitimate" diseases. Slowly, as more and more research gets published, the illness is baptized by having a diagnostic code assigned to it, included into the official and this, de-bastardized.

To be fair, CS is somewhere past the beginning phase of this normal process. A number of cases have been reported, and a number of peer reviewed articles have been published in respected journals. Concurrently, industry paid physicians and researchers publish articles that say CS is psychological, undermining efforts to legitimize CS as a non-psychological, physical condition. But, as of this writing, there has yet to be agreement as to the cause or underlying mechanisms of the disease. Given time, research and money, at some point, this situation should improve.[5]

It is also possible that CS is a politically incorrect ailment with a unique set of problems. As the middle name indicates, and as any PWCS will tell you, the culprit is a chemical. Yet, chemicals are basic to our industrial society. Full recognition of their health hazards, are financially threatening to very powerful interest groups. Even though producing a chemical that might cure CS, which is caused by chemicals, might be profitable to the industry, they have not been willing to do this.

This is particularly troublesome. According to an editorial on June 18, 2007 in *The New York Times*, the curriculum for continuing education courses, which all physicians are required to take in order to keep their medical knowledge on the cutting edge, have been subcontracted by the American Medical Association to the pharmaceutical industry.

Ignorance about this condition in the medical community is further compounded by the understandable skepticism of members of the profession, as well as the general public. It is difficult for an individual who is not chemically sensitive to accept the reality of the individual who is. Non-CS people, doctors included, use a multitude of chemical products daily. They are used, to name a few, for cleaning, personal hygiene, to kill pathogens, cover over unpleasant odors, and increase their sex appeal. They use them all the time, and they do not get sick. Attacking or blaming chemicals, which are perceived as an essential part of their life style, or for some, an essential part of their being, is foreign and unbelievable to them. Adopting the role model of the Ancient Greeks who killed the bearer of bad news, the non-CS person reacts with disbelief or even hostility to the

---

5. Some members of the CS community think that the chemical industry, with so much to lose if chemicals are proven hazardous to one's health has been blocking research into the illness and promoting the psychological causation theory.

PWCS who tries to explain that their deodorant, perfume, or what ever gets them sick.

It is also hypothesized that the powerful, pervasive advertising and marketing industries, the shapers of our current culture, further reinforce disbelief in CS. They have very effectively equated deodorants, fragrance, and fabric softeners with achieving success, love and community. Who has not seen the deodorant advertisement where a burley cave man type guy raises his arms, exposes his hairy armpits to a group of people who immediately fall into a stupor, overcome by his "natural" scent? Therefore, if you tell your CS doubting physician, who is a member of the official community as well as the culture, that chemicals, including the ones he is wearing, and clean his office with, make you sick, the most common response, said or thought, is that you must be crazy. The psychiatric community is about to make money, think they are going to make you better, while they probably make you sicker.

Reasons to Obtain an Accurate Differential Diagnosis and Receive Proper Treatment

As difficult and as frustrating as this task is, and although many PWCS have self-diagnosed themselves and obtained information about how to manage the illness from the internet, friends, or support groups, I believe it is helpful for most, and imperative for many, that one embarks on this difficult journey for the following reasons:

A qualified professional can rule out other conditions as the cause of the symptoms: There are many illnesses that have symptoms similar to CS. These include Lyme Disease, parasites, and neuropsychological disturbances. If the person does not have CS, they can receive treatment for the condition they actually do have. If they have CS, they may also have another condition that needs treatment with medications.

Some potentially overlapping disguised illnesses are treated with antibiotics (essentially chemicals that might make some PWCS ill and also disturb the normal intestinal flora creating an overgrowth of harmful yeast, which can also make one sick) for an extended period and that course of treatment may be life saving for some, but contraindicated for a chemically sensitive individual. Some alternative physicians might prescribe herbs or supplements, but although "natural" they too can make an individual ill.

By definition, Chemical Sensitivity means that the individual is sensitive to chemicals. All drugs are chemicals; even so called natural ones--think arsenic. Although some PWCS may be able to take various drugs without exacerbating their CS, there are innumerable ones that they cannot tolerate. In addition, one of the characteristics of this illness is that one can become sensitive to anything to which one is exposed to over a period of time. This obviously includes medications. The PWCS they could easily become sensitive to the medicine over time. Thus the magic bullet, intended to be therapeutic, might turn out to be the poison pill.

In the worst case scenario, as the good patient follows their doctor's recommendations, their CS progresses and their sensitivities increase and they become sensitive to a myriad of substances they were not sensitive to before undergoing treatment. If this happens they may get so sick that they may not even be able to travel to or tolerate the doctor's office to continue the treatment they were hoping would make them well. Thus, the well-meaning, but uninformed, physician, heroically trying to relieve the symptoms and suffering of his chemically sensitive patient using standard or unorthodox protocol, could be, because he does not understand the ramifications of this illness, inadvertently violating the Hippocratic Oath they took when their degree was presented to them. "Do no harm."

A qualified professional can validate the patient's reality and help them not feel "crazy": Being chemically sensitive is difficult, confusing, and is contrary to the norms of the current culture, therefore, it is important for the PWCS to understand what is happening to them and, that they are not crazy. Many individuals with this malady have consulted numerous physicians, at great expense, that have been unfamiliar with this illness and have had the reality of their experience of getting sick from chemicals disputed, or denied. Sometimes the professional assumes that the patient is a hypochondriac or is the physician is frustrated because he does not know what is going on and cannot hand the patient a prescription to fix it.

Some professionally challenged physician, rather than admit their lack of knowledge, or listen with an open mind in an attempt to get to the bottom of it, are tempted to tell the patient to "Take two aspirin" and hopefully forget to call in the morning. The physician that said this could not conceive that the supposedly innocuous coating the companies put on the aspirins to help people swallow them without leaving a bad taste in the mouth, or the color to make the pill look appetizing might get some PWCS sick.

Other professionals will reinforce the "You are crazy" theory by referring the patient to an equally chemically unaware member of the psychiatric community, a specialty which, often is given the job of medical waste basket. This is not helpful because CS is not a psychiatric illness, yet the CS unaware psychiatrist will do what they were trained to do, namely prescribe one psychotropic medication, see if it works, if not prescribe another. Often this is done in conjunction with psychotherapy, in the hopes that something will work.

The patient that goes this route can get sick in two ways: From undergoing psychotherapy in a potentially unsafe office; or from medication that cannot be tolerated by the PWCS. If the patient complains to the psychiatric professional about the air in the office, which might also include scented candles and or air fresheners, the psychiatrist is taught in "shrink school", as I was, to view this communication as "resistance to treatment", and will then proceed to investigate the "resistance," do cognitive therapy or clear up an internal thought distortion.

Obviously, even if there is no magic pill, having a respected qualified knowledgeable professional, label, explain, educate, and prescribe a treatment plan is affirming and reassuring to the confused sufferer. Knowing what is wrong with them and what their options are comforts most people. And needless to say, this approach protects them from further needless harm.

A qualified professional providing an accurate diagnosis will help a PWCS avoid unqualified practitioners and "quacks": The existence of an illness that has numerous, mysterious symptoms with no known cause, in a population that is desperate for relief from their suffering and frustrated with the failure of the orthodox medical community to help them, is fertile ground for the unethical practitioner. Admittedly, many alternative practitioners are well meaning, and some have been the only ones to correctly diagnose the condition. Some of their treatments might mitigate the symptoms, but others might make the patient worse. Yet unethical members of this less regulated community, or any of the other helping communities, may simply be in the financial strip mining business. Treatment with a member of this latter group often ends with either the patient getting worse, or not having enough resources to continue treatment. As a final insult, the practitioner might even blame the failure of the patient to get better on the patient for not following their prescribed protocol for a long enough period of time.

A qualified professional who validates the condition, respects the special needs of the PWCS. Obtaining understanding, support and cooperation from one's family and friends is a chronic problem for members of the CS community. Too often one's co-workers, spouse, children, parents, and/ or friends simply do not believe that the illness is real and feel imposed upon when asked not to wear scented products. They cannot understand why the PWCS claims they get sick from products that most people in the world use all the time without difficulty. Sometimes, the family and friends grow weary of the requests for accommodations and limitations being imposed on them. They think the patient should just get over it. Another problem is some people especially have linked their identity with a particular product. The result is defeat for the sufferer and victory for the marketer.

People within this mind-set sometimes interpret a request not to wear the product as "the person's racquet" or an attempt to control them, get sympathy or some other secondary gain. This reasoning is the same as that of the above mentioned physician, which is that the whole world uses these products and does not get sick, "What is wrong with you?" Others simply cannot be bothered and simply end the relationship. No wonder that the divorce rate among members of the CS community, as well as the suicide rate is very high. Most PWCS complain about a lack of support from family and friends.

While having a respected professional document the condition does not guarantee that the support system will stay in place, or the marital partner will honor their vows, it would nor hurt and certainly could help.

A qualified professional can guide the PWCS towards a new, healthier life. Acceptance by the PWCS of the ramifications of this illness is difficult. The life they once planned to live is over, never to fully return. Their pre-CS life and unfulfilled dreams are dead and have to be mourned. A new life, like the mythical Phoenix, has to be allowed to emerge from the ashes of the old. Another task is to learn to live with, and manage CS, but the learning curve is long. There is much to learn and much to change. There are no options. It must be done, and one's lifestyle altered to stop the *possible* downward degenerative spiral of this illness.

A correct diagnosis from a respected professional, an explanation of what is happening to you, and instructions on how to live a life that does not continue to make you sick or sicker are obviously the most important reasons to seek out such an individual. This is standard procedure with any serious illnesses, of which CS is one. There is life after contracting CS, but someone has to show you the right door to open and help you walk through it.

Finding a Specialist

Finding a qualified, and respected physician for this illness can be achieved in a number of ways. I suggest the following:

1. Start with the this book, which mentions the more well known specialists in this field.

2. Contact the Chemical Injury Information Network, (CIIN)[6] and request a referral list of practitioners and support groups for your area.

3. Talk to as many people as you can in the CS community, especially those in your area, to find out whom they use and what their experience has been. You could get lucky and find someone local. Sometimes, even the blind squirrel gets a nut.

4. Check with your local CS support group. If you do not know if there is one in your area, contact CIIN. They can supply you with a full referral list. Support groups usually have a list of local physicians qualified to treat the illness and hopefully, an evaluation of them.

5. Gather as much information you can about the prospective medical professional such as their fees, orientation and treatment methods.[7]

6. If you travel to see one of the specialists who is not within an acceptable distance from your home, make sure to ask about: the availability of lodging, food, costs, how long you have to stay there.

7. Find someone who has visited that particular specialist to find out what his or her experience has been.

8. Contact your local medical school or teaching hospital to find out if they have an environmental research facility that can treat or give you a referral.

---

6. 1-406-547-2255

7. The internet can offer help.

The Examination

It's best if the qualified professional conducts two concurrent examinations. The first is a standard, complete, physical examination to rule out the presence of any non-CS medical condition that has symptoms similar to those of CS or are concurrent with CS. A knowledgeable physician will go one step further to ascertain the level and types of chemical exposures you encounter in your daily life. The second exam, which could be done at the same time as the first, should include specific questions and tests to ascertain the possibility of chemical poisoning. A complete examination would include the following:

1. Detailed medical history and interview inquiring about possible:

    a. Genetic predisposition (family history and tests).

    b. Chemical exposure in the area in which you live.

    c. Chemicals in you household environment.

    d. Chemicals in the personal products you use.

    e. Chemicals in the work place.

    f. Chemicals in your diet, medications, or supplements.

    g. Existence of dental implants, and oral health status.

    h. Material that any fillings and bridges are made of.

    i. Other material that may have been implanted in the patient's body such as artificial hips, knees, pins, etc.

2. Presence of any infectious problems such as Lyme Disease, or others, which might have CS-like symptoms.

3. Checking for possible hormonal imbalances.

4. Examination of the cardio-circulatory system.

5. Evidence of skeletal muscular problems.

6. Testing for possible pollen, food, and dander allergies.

7. Stool analysis to look for parasites, infection, intestinal function, and/or presence of excessive amounts of yeast/Candida.

8. Eye, ear, nose, sinus and throat examination looking for any abnormalities or chronic infections.

9. Neurological examination to detect any non-CS neurological conditions such as tumors in the brain or nervous system as well as neurological damage or dysfunction that might be due to chemical poisoning.

10. Immune system functioning.

11. Vitamin and mineral levels.

12. Fatty acid levels.

13. Thyroid functioning.

14. Amino acid levels.

15. Antioxidant levels.

16. Specific tests to detect abnormal levels of toxic chemicals stored in the body such as solvents, petrochemicals, pesticides, and heavy metals.

17. Blood tests to detect the presence of chemicals and which ones are present.

18. Fatty tissue analysis for stored fat soluble chemicals in areas of the body where excess amounts are stored.

19. Examination of one's hair and nails to divulge chemicals.

If chemical poisoning is suspected from an analysis of the above information, many physicians confirm this, as well as to ascertain which chemicals are making the individual sick, by the following:

1. Chemical Challenge Tests: These are tests by which commonly offending, or suspected offending chemicals are introduced to the patient in various ways. They can be inhaled, put on the tongue or a small amount injected just under the skin. If the introduction of the chemical reproduces the symptom that the patient has presented, it is considered diagnostic, in other words, the patient is sensitive to that chemical. If they also react to a number of chemicals, they have Chemical Sensitivity. Also, through this test the physician can ascertain just how far the illness has progressed by the severity of the reaction to the challenge.

2. Neurological Testing: It is useful for treatment, and to

ascertain the seriousness of this condition to the patient and significant others, to assess the neurological damage that may have occurred due to a chemical injury. Neurological tests can include:

3. Questions about life style, diet, and other items should be a part of your environmental screening.

A. Balance tests.

B. Reflex tests.

C. Finding any areas in the brain that may be damaged through a PET, SPECT scans and/or a QEEG.

D. Neuropsychological and cognitive functioning tests will show any damage to the cognitive area of the brain, and if and how it has affected brain functioning.

Arriving at a Diagnosis of CS

Even though there is no single definitive, testable, commonly accepted and clinically replicated marker, an analysis of all the above should indicate if the patient has CS or not, and disclose what, if any, damage due to toxic chemical exposure was found.

There are no universally accepted diagnostic criteria for CS as there are for other diseases that lack a specific marker or test. Most PWCS self-diagnose because they know that chemical exposures make them ill.

Thus, CS is a diagnosis of exclusion, with all other possible diseases ruled out, combined with the observable reaction of the patient to chemicals. The physician, having conducted the examination and arriving at a diagnosis of CS, will explain the illness to the individual and recommend a treatment plan. Treatment will be discussed in a subsequent chapter.

Receiving an accurate diagnosis, based on thorough physical examinations by a qualified professional, should start to alleviate the PWCS's suffering, validate their experience and help them (not guaranteed due to the nature of this condition) with any doubting friends and relatives.

What To Do if There is No "Expert" in Your Area

You may live too far from the nearest expert or may simply need a relatively aware and flexible physician for your non-CS, normal medical needs. The next best thing is to find a physician in your area with some experience with CS or at least one who will be open to the possibility of chemical injury and willing to learn about it.

This is important for three reasons: The physician may be willing to consult with a physician who is more knowledgeable, and learn and thus be able to treat you; The physician may be able to help treat the illness using published, established CS protocols; If you are hospitalized, the physician may be able to make your stay easier by acting as an advocate for you with the hospital staff. The local physician's degree of knowledge and flexibility will obviously vary, but some knowledge is better than none. Flexibility and openness are highly valued and information in this internet era is readily available.

In the absence of an expert or experienced physician, is a physician who, although not familiar with CS, has at least heard of it, and is not prejudiced against believing in it. This physician may be willing to learn about it or give you a referral to a more specifically knowledgeable health care professional.

If you must use a physician who has never heard of this condition, don't try to immediately educate her or him on all aspects of CS unless you want to drive the physician away or be driven away with a referral to a psychiatrist.

A better strategy is to build your relationship on non-CS health concerns over a long period. This will bond the physician to you, and gradually invest her/him in your health. Over time, slowly introduce some of the CS related problems you are having. If you get a negative result after this careful procedure, find another physician.

Cautions

It is best to be familiar with the results of the various surveys that have been done on the effectiveness of various treatments in order to make an informed cost/effectiveness decision as to any doctor's treatment recommendations.[8]

---

8. See the survey in the appendix and the full Gibson Survey in; *M.C.S. a Survival Guide.*

Beware of the physician, who claims to be able to treat this condition and actually thinks he or she does, but does not. Unfortunately treatment from this type of health practitioner has four possible negative outcomes: It can often make you worse; cost a lot of money; waste a lot of time; increase your frustration/anger level. All of these may not help you become healthy.

The medical health professionals, who view a desperate population with an incurable disease who have not been helped by the orthodox medical community, as a potential gold mine to prospect, are the ones to especially look out for. They give you false hope by promising to cure you with this or that product, treatment plan, or device. During the treatment process they raise your hopes and lower your financial resources. When you complain that you are getting worse, many will say, "That is great. It shows the treatment is working. You have to get worse, before you get better."

What to Look For In a Doctor If You Can't Find a CS Specialist

When seeing an unknown doctor for the first time, and you have to make your own judgment as to the quality of care you will receive, I suggest the following check lists. Obviously, only an expert that specializes in CS will fulfill all or most of the following, but fulfilling some of the requirements is better than nothing and gives an indication as to how sensitive the physician is to this condition.

I. Office and physical surroundings:

A. Toxicity: A capable physician, familiar with CS should have a nontoxic, odor free office that represents an understanding of the problem. Specifically that means:

1. Well offgassed hardwood or tiled floor without synthetic carpets or rugs.

2. The air in the office and waiting room should be filtered, and not have a smell.

3. A vestibule or some other chamber to separate the waiting room and office from the outside.

4. A location in the least toxic part of town, preferably on a side street upwind of any industry or highway traffic.

5. The office should not share a building with a toxin emitting. commercial firm such as dry cleaners, candle store, fragrance shop, photo processing lab, or any other such business.

6. The office should be fragrance, food, and newsprint free, with signs posted to that effect. No air fresheners.

7. No vegetation present in the office, as it can produce mold and pollen.

8. No ozone machines.

9. No patients or guests wearing fragrance are allowed in.

10. Nontoxic, safe lodging should be available for out of town, very sensitive patients.

11. If the office is in a high rise, it is best to be located downwind of elevators and stairwells, as they act as chimneys, bringing in toxins and other substances from the basement and other tenants.

II. Staff:

I tend to partially judge the physician by the quality of the office staff. I go under the assumption that having a good staff, which was most likely hired by the physician, shows some attention to detail as they are the first point of contact with a patient and therefore, represent and reflect the physician.

A. Staff should be fragrance free.

B. Staff should be pleasant and helpful.

C. It is best if the hands-on staff wears lab coats, and if bending over you to take blood or test for allergy, have a cap covering their hair.

D. Staff should be knowledgeable and willing to talk about any procedure or testing they are doing.

III. Physician:

A. The more specialties the physician has, the better. Look for, not necessarily in any order of importance, the following: Allergy, Environmental Medicine, Clinical Ecology, Emergency Medicine, Immunology, Occupational Medicine, Industrial Medicine, Internal Medicine, Neurology, Public Health, and Toxicology.

B. The physician should be familiar with all of the different theories and approaches to the illness, and be willing and able to discuss them with you.

C. The physician should share the chances of success and cost\ effectiveness of any treatment suggested with you.

D. The physician or a knowledgeable substitute should be on call during the business hours, or have available a knowledgeable substitute in case you have an emergency or a severe reaction to any test or treatment. It is not fun to be sick after office hours, possibly from the test or treatment, call the physician and reach an answering machine referring you to 911 or the local hospital. It is unlikely they would be able to offer you the specialized assistance you need from the doctor treating you.

E. The physician might be able to refer you to an "environmental unit" at a school or hospital that specializes in diagnosing and treating CS.

F. The physician should have hospital admitting privileges at a local hospital that is CS friendly, even if they are not expert, so that the your CS special needs can be met as well as possible.

G. The physician should have available referrals to knowledgeable health care practitioners for specialized tests if needed.

H. The physician should be aware of any support groups in the area and be willing to refer you to them.

I. The physician should personally take, or ask for, a detailed medical history including possible toxins you have been exposed to, life style, diet, and other items that would part of your environmental screening.

J. Obvious danger signs to watch for in the medical candidate:

   1.   Too quick to prescribe prescription medication.

   2.   Suggestion to take a psychotropic drug or see a psychiatrist.

   3.   "Try my treatment and you will be cured in x period of time."

   4.   When complaining that the treatment is making you worse, having the physician tell you that you have to get worse to get better.

   5.   You are feeling worse because of "yeast die off" and you

should continue. This could be a sign of toxic overload caused by toxins being released by the dying yeast and indicate treatment should be slowed down.

6. Walking out of the office carrying a shopping bag filled with vitamins, herbs, minerals and other such ingredients, which, if needed, can be purchased much cheaper at a pharmacy or health food store.

7. Diagnosing the cause of your CS without testing to confirm it.

IV. Flexibility of the Physician:

A. If the office is environmentally OK but not perfect, you might ask to be the first appointment of the day so that you do not have to wait too long in an environment that might contain people wearing fragrance and the noxious fragrance residue of people and procedures that preceded you. Having a flexible office that will comply with your request is essential.

B. A flexible physician will be willing to read literature you provide or consult with one of the specialists in the field.

C. A flexible physician will be willing to consider the concerns you raise on the basis of your CS in regards to any treatment or medication under consideration without considering you uncooperative or non-compliant.

Obviously any health practitioner in possession of all of the above is most likely impossible to find at present. However, fulfilling some of the requirements is certainly better than none. I also recognize that given the current state of American medicine and the increasing control that the insurance industry has over the profession, it is getting more difficult for even the best doctors to spend the amount of time necessary to fulfill all of the above requirements, and many may have to return back to the time when a physician was also the pharmacist, and barber to earn a living.

Finding a Dentist that Understands CS

Finding a dentist familiar with sensitivities is even a more daunting task than finding a CS medical specialist. It is also fraught with more dangers. The number of dentists that are familiar with CS is even smaller than the number of knowledgeable doctors. It might even be more necessary to find one close by. If you have an abscess in the middle of the night, you cannot get on an airplane and travel 1000 miles to your environmental dentist. In addition, dental offices are notoriously toxic due to the materials that they use, a lab on the premise, and the amount of electrical equipment they need.

The danger is that the term "holistic dentistry" has become a profitable catchword. Unqualified "holistic dentists" and "mercury removers" abound. What may be holistic for the average dental patient and profitable for the dentist is most likely toxic for the PWCS. Improper removal of mercury fillings can be quite dangerous to the chemically sensitive individual, as well as the dentist.

Other obvious dangers of having dental work done, aside from the physical office, are: anesthesia that has to be injected to dull pain during a procedure; the material comprising the filling, bridge, cap, root canal, implant, and the adhesives used; or dentures which will live in your mouth for a long, long time.

Many so called environmental dentists advertise dental compatibility tests to learn about which materials their patient will tolerate. Although some individuals have found this valuable, many have not. In this illness, as mentioned above, a PWCS can become sensitive to anything that they come in contact with for an extended period of time. Just the fact that you did not react to a certain material at the time of the test, does not guarantee that you will not become sensitized to it at a later date after it has been permanently installed in your mouth.

What's a Poor Patient to Do?

There are no good answers that work for everyone. However, there are rules of thumb, most of them are common sense that comes from understanding CS:

1. Try and find a dentist who is familiar with this illness and has had experience. If you are lucky, that dentist can competently guide you through the dental work you need.

2. Find this dentist by the same methods you went looking for a medical doctor—word of mouth, support groups, etc.

3. If the dentist's orientation is an unknown quantity, apply as many of the rules for evaluating a physician as possible with

the expectation that the average dentist will fall far short of the desired ideal.

4. Interview the dentist you are considering to see the depth and breathe of his understanding of CS and flexibility.

5. Learn as much as you can about dental materials available and opt for the most inert ingredients possible for any filling, cap, or appliance. Success has generally been reported with porcelain for caps, bridges, and even fillings.

6. Stay away from anything with metal in it. This includes gold, no matter its purity. Metal, usually gold or steel, is used to strengthen large bridges; however, the same appliance can be made of zirconium, which is nontoxic for most, but is expensive and must be made by a specialty lab.

7. Filling materials might be needed.

    a. Many people tolerate synthetic fillings; others can only tolerate porcelain made in a lab from a mold.

    b. If you are electromagnetically sensitive, the lights, drills, and laser gun used to cement fillings in place will give you trouble.[9]

    c. A safe adhesive can only be found by trial and error. Fortunately adhesives offgass and become inert under the tooth.

8. Implants and root canals have gotten a mixed review from the community. For implants, titanium is the preferred material, and some PWCS have tolerated it. Others have had to have them removed, a nasty process as they are imbedded deep in the jaw. A great looking mouth and preservation of your original teeth may have to be sacrificed to the CS deity.

9. Surprisingly, some synthetic dental materials used for bridges and plates can be tolerated by many members of this community. The working rule is the harder and more inert the material, the better.

---

9. I personally do not know a way out of this and would appreciate it if any of the readers of this work would contact me if they have found a solution to this problem.

10. Your initial tolerance for anesthesia products can be determined for with a scratch test such as an allergist would use.

11. It is best to use anesthesia that does not contain ANY preservative or adrenalin. Preservative free Lidocaine is a good option.

12. Many PWCS can tolerate nitrous oxide, "laughing gas", as a mild anesthetic, thus bypassing the need for a Novocaine-like substance for minor procedures.

13. Nitrous leaves the system quickly and will clear even quicker if oxygen is administered afterwards, as well as during. However, the facemask used in its delivery might be a problem for some.

14. Acupuncture works as an anesthesia for many people if you can find a dental practitioner who is also a trained acupuncturist, or bring one in.

15. Latex gloves should NEVER be used even if you are not latex sensitive, as repeated exposure may produce severe latex sensitivity, which is not nice. Think of how often you encounter latex, during your normal day: toll collectors, gloves on food handlers, catheters, etc.

16. If you are having your teeth cleaned, request pure pumice to avoid any coloring or flavoring agents that might contain materials which might get one sick.

17. New appliances work best if they are soaked in a solution of baking soda for a day or so to remove any residue of the manufacturing process before being used in one's mouth.

18. Any appliance that has an odor after extensive soaking should not be allowed in your mouth until it is odor free.

19. As a last resort, (although a probably inaccurate test as the dental material will be in your mouth for a longer time), take home a piece of the proposed dental material and hold it in your mouth, between your gum and cheek, for as long a time as possible and note any reaction. You can even have a small ball of the adhesive made and test it the same way before it is permanently cemented in your mouth.

20. Some people choose to remove their mercury amalgam fillings, hoping it will improve their health, but this is a tough call. The Gibson survey that reports that 47% of those questioned reported no noticeable effect after removing the amalgam fillings. However what the long term effect on the health of those that had them removed and the mercury levels in the body was not noted. [10]

   a. There is potential danger is leaving them in, and danger in the removal process.

   b. If not removed properly by an experienced dentist, you could breathe in the vaporized mercury that occurs during the process. Some members of the community believe that you should leave sleeping dogs lie. Others are just as adamant on the other side.

   c. Yet, the American Dental Society maintains that mercury amalgam is nontoxic.

21. If you decide to remove your mercury fillings, make sure that the dentist is thoroughly familiar with the process. It is very important that the dentist puts a dam that you can tolerate in your mouth, an oxygen mask on your nose, and one on his nose. This will lessen the danger to both of you from inhaling mercury fumes.

With information, hard work, luck, and tact one can successfully navigate the medical and dental communities.

---

10. Mercury is a known poison that is stored in the body and difficult to eliminate. However, the American Dental Association deems mercury amalgam fillings safe. They argue that it is no longer pure mercury as it has been amalgamated with silver, another toxin, and supposedly has changed the composition of both. This is not logical. The mercury/silver amalgam sitting in a lab, doing nothing may indeed be inert, but what happens when it is subjected to the chewing and grinding motion that goes on in a normal mouth? In addition, dentists using mercury have to carefully, under supervision, according to strict toxic substance disposal rules, dispose of any and all excess filling material in a prescribed way. The mercury in one's mouth also leaches off slowly into the system as you chew food and vaporize the mercury in the top surface of the filling. Why would anyone want something permanently in his or her mouth that cannot be thrown in the garbage or down a toilet?

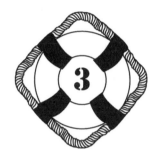

Treatment Options

There are many treatments for Chemical Sensitivity, but as of this writing, no cure. These treatments are designed to alleviate symptoms and help the body heal as much as possible. The degree of success varies, and depends on innumerable factors. Among these are: the extent to which the disease has progressed; the specific toxin that has assaulted the body; and the resiliency of the injured individual's system. This chapter will discuss the more popular treatments, their reported effectiveness, and the theories used to justify them.

Before one embarks on a treatment that might be expensive and time consuming, it is advisable to review the experience of other PWCS, and which treatments they have used and what their success has been. Fortunately, three surveys of treatments and their effectiveness on PWCS have been compiled which tabulate the self reported effectiveness of over 100 different treatments tried on a population base of almost one thousand chemically sensitive individuals.[1]

---

1. Although limited as they are based on self-reported data, they are the only guide available as to which of the reported treatments are most effective. Even more important they include which ones

There are several factors to consider before deciding on a treatment:

1. Is the reported success of the treatment worth the time and money necessary to do it?

2. Is the risk that the treatment might make one worse worth taking?

3. Does one have the financial resources to sustain the treatment for its expected length?

4. Is the treatment or facilities necessary to administer it readily available?

5. Is one's philosophical view of life congruent with the treatment?

At first glance the reported success of the various treatments is discouraging. Yet, before one falls down the well of hopelessness, it should be noted that even if only 15% of the respondents reported success, those 15% were helped. Therefore, a treatment with a favorable risk to reward ratio might be worth a try. As the advertisement for the New York Lottery says, "You never know."

The most accepted theory of this illness is that chemicals have overwhelmed and damaged the natural detoxification mechanisms of the body. Therefore, the now chemically sensitive individual gets sick from chemicals because their system has difficulty detoxifying from a chemical exposure. Then, the un-excreted chemicals that were inhaled, ingested, and/or absorbed, find their way to the brain and can cause neurological damage.

In many cases the overburdened detoxification system valiantly struggles to keep the individual safe by walling off excess chemicals in the fatty tissues of the body. This is only a temporary solution as these chemicals leach into the blood, and some can cross the blood brain barrier.

Many physicians try to solve this problem by recommending as

---

are reported to cause harm. Even with their limitations, they should be consulted before one in vests a lot of time and money on a suggested or prescribed treatment. They are: LeRoy Davis, and Jason, "Treatment Efficacy: A Survey of 305 MCS Patients" *The CFIDS Chronicle, Winter, 1996; Johnson,* "Survey Results from 351 Respondents," September 19, 1997, Brunswick, Maine, Alison Johnson; Gibson, Pamela, "Self Reported Treatment Efficacy in 917 Persons with Chemical Sensitivity," *Chemical Sensitivity: A Survival Guide*, Churchville, VA; Earthrive Books, 2006. It is certainly possible that many individuals engaged in all three surveys so the total number of respondents in not known. An abreviated version is in the appendix of this book.

much avoidance as possible and mechanically, nutritionally, and pharmaceutically supporting whatever detoxification mechanisms are still functioning. The most important organ in the body for detoxification is the liver and many physicians recommend treatments that support detoxification and liver function.

The Following Are Some Of The Treatments PWCS Have Tried:

Avoidance of Chemicals and Substances that Cause Reactions:

Over 94% of those surveyed reported feeling better and gradual improvement, by avoiding chemical exposure. Avoidance is defined to include: a chemical free living space, especially the bedroom; using nontoxic personal care and cleaning products; ability to work in a chemically free work environment; and eating chemically free, organic food, rather than food grown with chemicals and containing potentially harmful additives.

There are obvious difficulties practicing avoidance. Complete avoidance of chemicals in the 21st Century is easier to say than do. As simple a matter as finding clean air to breathe in the United States is becoming more and more difficult each year. Even in states with notoriously bad air, there are less toxic places to live, as well as microenvironments that can be found. The issue is not only whether they exist, but, locating them. As much as the CS community needs it, a central information agency to help find this type of sanctuary, unfortunately does not exist. In addition, published information on the toxicity of various places such as that supplied by the EPA and on www. scorecard.org, is most likely out of date and does not cover all substances that various individuals are sensitive to. Everyone is different. What bothers one person might not bother another. Furthermore, all geographic areas have problems, and moving entails psychological as well as financial stress.

In some cases this seemingly hopeless task might have to be attempted. There are serious dangers in remaining in a known toxic environment. Certain chemicals destroy brain cells and CS is a progressive illness. When it progresses, the individual becomes sensitive to more and more substances, and in smaller concentrations. The end point of this degenerative process can be severe total disability. In addition, there can be the danger of major organ failure. Therefore, if you are living in an environment containing substances that make you sick, it behooves you to find a less toxic place in which to live and work

Cleaning Up Your Current Environment:

Before one runs to a fantasy safe place to live, which might prove to be worse than the one left, one should attempt to make the place in which one is living as clean as possible.[2] The first step to cleaner air and better health is to identify and remove all toxic items from your home and replace them with those that do not make you sick. The second step is to repeat the process with your personal care products. The third step, if one and two have not helped sufficiently, is to determine if the structure of your home is good enough in order that it can be made safer. This later step is additionally dependent upon the outside air and area in which your home is located.

Even if the outside air is not so bad or good enough, living in a toxic house that cannot be made safe is certainly not advised. Air filters may help, but they will not save you, despite the claims of the filter manufactures claim, and many sufferers hope. Inside air cannot be made appreciably better than the outside air unless one has unlimited resources to install a "space shuttle quality" air filtration device.

It must be seriously noted that all of the respected treatment plans even those with the greatest reported chances of success are strictly predicated on the requirement that the individual undergoing the treatment has a clean place in which to live, practices avoidance, and uses nontoxic cleaning and personal care products. Even if you undergo a successful course of treatment at a respected treatment center, feel better, and then return to the same "toxic" environment from whence you came, the benefits will shortly disappear.

Creating a Chemically Free Oasis in Which to Live and Sleep:

Obviously a PWCS will feel better in a chemically free environment, which in which their body is not under constant toxic assault. Living in such a place allows the body to rest, utilize, and repair detoxification systems that are not permanently broken.

The human body contains mechanisms to heal damage to systems that are not broken beyond repair. These mechanisms can best be helped in this illness by exposing the system to the least amount of environmental and psychological assaults. If the body does not have to use up its resources

---

2. A more complete discussion of what to look for in choosing a new place to live, whether or not to move, fixing up an existing house, and nontoxic cleaning as well as personal care products will be discussed in other chapters of this work.

fighting new, continued chemical insults, it will have more available energy to eliminate stored toxins (detoxify) and repair as much of the damage as it can.

The degree to which one gets better will depend on the usual suspects: genetics; type of exposure; degree of injury; and the level of a toxic free environment. Since roughly one-third of one's life is spent sleeping, the bedroom is the most important room in which to set up a safe oasis to feel better in and help the body eliminate stored chemicals.

A great majority of people report feeling better with this method, and many have even been able to regain some portion of their previous life. Yet, to accomplish the later is a slow process. In a long journey without landmarks, progress is difficult to note, and discouragement easy. Counteract this human tendency to drift into negative thinking by keeping a daily log of how you are feeling in order to compare your progress against previous periods. If you get discouraged it might be helpful to remember that we are the latest survivors in a long human chain. To have accomplished this, systems evolved that allowed the human race to overcome all sorts of chemical and biological insults. History proves that our systems are remarkably resilient. Trust it. If allowed to rest and repair in an environment where it does not have to exhaust itself fighting repeated toxic assaults, the body will do its best to right itself.

Detoxification:

There are numerous ways to detoxify the body from toxic material. Some of the more popular ones will be discussed in this section.

Sauna Detoxification:

Saunas and heat therapy have been used by innumerable cultures for centuries to detoxify the human body and promote health. Well known examples are: Finnish Saunas, Turkish Baths, Russian Baths, and Native American Sweat Lodges. Exposing the system to heat mechanically helps the detoxification system by forcing the individual to "sweat" many stored and newly acquired toxins out of the body and on to the skin where they can be washed down the drain.

Sauna, or more accurately "heat chamber detoxification" assumes a nontoxic sauna, chemically free water in which to wash afterwards, nontoxic soap to cleanse the skin, replacement of any lost fluids, minerals and Vitamins, and regular intestinal transit time, as some toxins are eliminated through the alimentary canal.

Any type of heat will work. Some individuals report successful detoxification by exercising to work up a sweat in a chemically free place such as a beach or desert. This is obviously the least expensive method if one lives in such an area.

Dry heat in a nontoxic sauna, or heat chamber, is the most commonly used method, although many people have experienced relief by soaking in a bathtub containing various salts or minerals, or in a steam bath. The latter two are not methods of choice unless dry heat is not available. The danger of wet heat is that during the process of soaking, the water will soon contain excreted chemicals. These can be reabsorbed through the heated and thus more porous skin, the largest organ in the body.

A sauna detoxification program can be done under medical supervision at one of the specialized treatment centers in the United States, such as the Environmental Health Center of Dallas, Texas or The Center for Occupational and Environmental Medicine in North Charleston, South Carolina. A home sauna, using a less stringent protocol if direct medical supervision is not available, will also work if care is taken, and a physician, after an evaluation of your general health approves of it.

A. Professional Sauna Detoxification:

As noted, sauna detoxification therapy is routinely offered at the specialized treatment centers in the United States. Physicians at these centers usually recommend a 4-6 week program, usually consisting of three treatments a day. The following are variations of a sauna protocol developed by L. Ron Hubbard to detoxify drug addicts, and modified by various environmental physicians.[3]

1. Twenty minutes of aerobic exercise to mobilize the chemicals stored in the body.

2. 1000 mg. of oral Vitamin C to oxidize the chemicals that the heat will release into the blood stream.

3. 20 minutes in the sauna at 120-140 degrees. Some PWCS will have to build up to this slowly. Others may have to stay

---

3. L. Ron Hubbard, *Clear Body Clear Mind: The Effective Purification Program*, CA: Bridge Publications, 1990. Hubbard also noted that when he put recovering drug addicts in a sauna they would often re-experience the "highs" of the drugs that they had taken, and often, oily, smelly, substances exuded from their bodies. Some PWCS report that saunas made them worse--perhaps for the same reason.

in longer, in order to sweat. If one has difficulty sweating, exercising before or while in the sauna is recommended.

4. An immediate shower in chlorine free filtered water to rinse the chemicals off of the skin.[4]

5. Another 1000 mg. dose of Vitamin C.

6. One ounce of vegetable oil ingested orally. The rational for doing this is that the body will replace the bad fats containing chemicals with good and also slow down any possible re-absorption via the gastrointestinal tract.

7. A half a teaspoonful of Tri-Salts® which contain calcium, potassium and magnesium to replace any of these vital electrolytes lost during the treatment.

8. Ingest ¼ of a teaspoonful of potassium chloride for the same reason.

9. A multi-mineral capsule to replace any which might have been lost during the treatment.

10. A massage to mobilize the chemicals out of the fatty tissues.

11. At the Environmental Health Center of Dallas the process is repeated two more times during the day. (L. Ron Hubbard recommends a much longer time in the sauna with a buddy to guard against problems from over exposure, and a more extensive Vitamin and mineral regimen.)

12. A weekly blood test should be done to insure that the electrolyte balance of the body has not been compromised.

The main disadvantages of this treatment are: cost, distance from a treatment center, breathing in and thus absorbing the excreted toxins of other individuals who might be in the sauna with you, and returning home to a toxic environment where the benefits will be lost, as the basic problem, that of a broken detoxification system, have not been solved.

---

4. Use cold or cool water to lessen the chances of chemicals on the skin being reabsorbed into the body.

B. Home Sauna:

Instead of going to a treatment center, a home sauna unit, of which many are available, can be purchased or built. The most recommended commercial sauna is made of kiln dried poplar wood and glass, heated by a sauna heater, and vented. Numerous brands are available from such sources as 1-800-MySauna; or the Environmental Health Foundation of Dallas.

One has a choice between a standard sauna and one that emits infrared heat. At present, there is not enough data available to determine if the newer infrared saunas are any more effective, as claimed, than the standard one. If one is EMF sensitive, infrared saunas are said to be better. But a standard sauna can be heated to the proper temperature, and then turned off before the EMF sensitive individual enters--thus the benefits of heat with no exposure to an electromagnetic field.

The problem with a wood sauna is that over time the wood absorbs some of the excreted chemicals and thus obtains and emits an odor, possibly toxic. Sanding the top layer of the wood when it starts to smell can eliminate this. An advantage of a commercial wood sauna is that if one moves, the sauna can easily be easily disassembled and reassembled in a new location using only simple tools.

An alternative is to construct a ceramic sauna, or more accurately a heat chamber.[5] To create one, simply install a sauna heater in an insulated closet that has been covered with ceramic tile. For a heater one can use either an infrared or regular one that can be obtained from one of the numerous sources such as Finlandia. Add lights to read by, a ceramic bench to sit or lie on, a glass door, easily purchased or installed by a glass company, through which to watch TV from, and an exhaust fan to clear the toxins which will be emitting from your body, out of the chamber. To pass the time, one can meditate, write, read a book, or watch television through the glass door of the sauna. TV sound can be heard by running an offgassed computer speaker from the headphone jack on the television set into or near the sauna.

Public saunas such as those provided by health clubs are not recommended. They are usually too hot. Most environmental physicians recommend that the sauna be heated to 120-140 degrees, which is much less than a commercial sauna, which can be as high as 200 degrees. Another problem is

---

5. Traditional saunas enthusiasts claim that it has to be made of wood to be called a sauna. For a fuller discussion of the benefits of sauna for PWCS and how to construct a home sauna, see: Marilyn G. McVicker, *Sauna Detoxification Therapy*, North Carolina: McFarland & Co. Publishers, 1997.

that other individuals use them who are more likely than not have odiferous substances emitting from their bodies for you to inhale. In addition, the saunas are cleaned with strong toxic antiseptic chemicals given their public availability. Public saunas are also fragrant, either from the wood used or something that the management adds to counteract body odors.

If one chooses to undergo home sauna therapy, a variation of the above treatment center's protocol can be used. Usually less frequent treatment is recommended as well as a local medical doctor's approval. Electrolyte levels can easily be checked with a standard blood test ordered by any physician.

As a cautionary note—when one starts sauna therapy for the first time there might be a tendency to feel worse while in the sauna. This is because previously stored chemicals are being released into the blood stream. The symptoms clear up as the body starts to sweat and detoxify. There might also be mood changes while one is in the heat chamber, as the chemicals released from the tissues can affect the brain's neurotransmitters, which control moods. This may be the reason that 15% of individuals who have tried sauna therapy report that the therapy was harmful to them. If in doubt, check with a physician.

To reiterate, sauna treatments do not have any lasting effect if one is still living or working in a toxic environment.

A third precaution is obviously anyone embarking on a sauna detoxification program should only do so with his or her doctor's approval.

Other Detoxification Methods:

Innumerable other health practitioners recommend various pharmaceuticals, herbs, nutrients, and mechanical procedures on the theory that they help the detoxification mechanisms of the liver, gall bladder, and bowel. These include such procedures as coffee enemas, bowel cleansers, colonics, applying external heat to the liver, and Eastern Medicine techniques. Before one embarks on an expensive and time consuming course of therapy either self-directed or under the advice of a health care practitioner, this book suggests that you consult the afore mentioned surveys as to their reported effectiveness/harm ratio before embarking on what might be a long and expensive course of treatment.

The results of these treatments vary and can be found in the previously mentioned treatment surveys. It should be noted that Dr. Pamela Gibson reports that "40 percent of the research participants who tried coffee enemas and 35 percent of those who experimented with bowel cleanses rated them as having great benefit."[6] Yet about 20 percent of the individuals using coffee enemas and gallbladder flushes reported that they were harmful, as well as 12 percent of those using bowel cleansers. This is another example of a risk reward decision that one has to make when deciding upon a treatment for CS.

A. Supporting the Liver:

The liver is the major detoxification organ in the human body and needs various Vitamins, minerals and nutrients or order to function most efficiently. Specialized blood tests can determine their levels in the body, and if found deficient, they can be added to the diet in the form of supplements. A qualified practitioner should do this. The most commonly prescribed and most important ingredient for best liver functioning is the amino acid, glutathione. Unfortunately the acid and digestive juices in the stomach deactivate orally ingested glutathione. Many practitioners attempt to avoid this by administering it intravenously along with other nutrients.

Other environmental physicians recommend self-administering glutathione two to four times a day by oral inhalation. To counteract any sensitivity due to inflamed lungs, they recommend building up tolerance slowly to a therapeutic dose contained in 2 ml. of buffered preservative free diluents. They generally start with one drop of glutathione in two ml. of distilled water. Some also add hydroxycobalamine, a form of Vitamin B12 which they claim has the effect of reducing neural inflammation. They also recommend an assortment of Vitamins, minerals, and other substances, which they argue are necessary for the glutathione to be most effective. [7]

The amounts and quantities of these Vitamins, oils, enzymes, and minerals are obtained from extensive laboratory blood and saliva tests. The later supplements are administered orally. They also recommend nasal inhalation of glutathione and hydroxycobalamine to counteract acute chemical exposures.

At present there are only anecdotal reports as to the effectiveness of

6. Gibson, Pamela, "Self Reported Treatment Efficacy in 917 Persons with Chemical Sensitivity," *Chemical Sensitivity: A Survival Guide*, Churchville, VA; Earthrive Books, 2006. p.12.

7. For a fuller discussion of this see Dr. Grace Ziem's discussion of "neural sensitivity" and her treatment plan at: http://www.chemicalinjury.net.htm

this approach. In addition, it is expensive, and the patient is asked to make a two year commitment to the treatment. Of the few people that I have talked to, some say it helped immensely, others said it had no effect, and still others dropped out due to the high cost.

If oral inhalation of glutathione cannot be tolerated due to lung irritation, these physicians still recommend it, but as a nasal spray. Oral ingestion of glutathione is not recommended as the stomach acid destroys the drug. Obviously, alcohol should not be used by people with CS.

B. Intravenous Therapy to Detoxify and Support General Health:

Many practitioners that specialize in CS recommend a course of intravenous (IV) therapy. 1-3 times a week a PWCS allows administration, by a slow drip, of a preservative free solution, from a glass, not plastic bottle. The IV contains high doses of Vitamin C, plus minerals, and glutathione. The theory is that the body is deficient in the Vitamins and minerals, and replacing them with an IV, bypassing the stomach that might not be able to absorb necessary nutrients, is the best way to help the PWCS regain health. Glutathione has been discussed earlier as a liver support; and high mega doses of Vitamin C are thought to "burn off" the chemicals in the blood stream. Although widely used by environmental physicians, success rates have not been tabulated for this form of treatment and anecdotal reports are mixed.

A disadvantage is the cost, up to $115-$225 per treatment as of this writing. However, if cost is not a factor, the individual is not sensitive to the ingredients, which can be ascertained via a skin test, and the treatment is administered in a nontoxic environment using chemically free substances that the individual does not react to, in glass rather than plastic containers, and using a metal rather than a plastic needle, there is little potential harm.

Before one embarks on this treatment, it is recommended that Vitamin, mineral, and glutathione levels be checked to see if they are adequate or deficient.

C. Oxygen Therapy:

Many environmental physicians recommend inhaled oxygen to counteract an acute attack and recommend that their patients keep a tank of oxygen in their homes at all times. The individual is instructed to use it during an extreme attack, and sometimes recommended for a period of each day over a long period of time.

The reasoning behind this is that oxygen supposedly "burns up" chemicals in the blood stream and since chemical exposure decreases the brain's oxygen supply, inhaled oxygen counteracts it. Oxygen also helps counteract any oxygen depletion in the brain that might be caused by a chemical exposure.

Oxygen for chemical exposure is not normally covered by insurance, but it is not that expensive. Since 70% of those surveyed report that the procedure was helpful, oxygen is well worth having in case of an emergency. Some individuals even keep a small tank of oxygen in their vehicle to counteract road fumes. A small size container is also available and that could be kept with you at all times in case of emergency.

The normal recommended dose of oxygen is 2-3 ml per hour. More is not recommended as it can interfere with the lung functioning. Some people experience difficulty with the plastic tubing and nasal canella that is normally supplied by the oxygen company. To counteract this if at all possible, do not use the canella fresh out of the package. Obtain one well in advance of when it is needed, soak it in solution of baking soda and give it time to offgass. Preparing a spare is strongly advised.

If the plastic canella still bothers you, Tygon™ tubing that is less toxic, as well as a ceramic mask can be purchased from numerous sources such as the American Environmental Health Foundation.

D. Hyperbaric Oxygen Treatments:

This involves the person entering a specialized chamber that looks similar to an enclosed tanning machine and having it filled with oxygen at two to three times the atmospheric pressure at sea level for one hour a day for approximately thirty days. It is believed that the increased pressure forces the oxygen into all the tissues of the body which then forces out and oxidizes stored toxins. This form of treatment has been used for years for acute chemical poisoning as well as for deep-sea divers who have gotten the "bends." It has also shown effectiveness in many non-CS conditions. Although its effectiveness for CS has been favorably anecdotally reported, a judgement cannot be made as the treatment evolved after the surveys were taken and tabulated.

The disadvantages of hyperbaric oxygen treatment are: the cost tends to be high, ($100-$300 per treatment depending on where you live) and generally not covered by insurance policies; the length of time needed; the availability of a facility that has a chamber; and the chemically free nature of such a facility and unit. The later can be partially helped by bringing one's own sheets to buffer you from the material in the hyperbaric oxygen unit.

Treatments Based on the Immunological Model:

Even though discounted by the current group of researchers, many environmental physicians believe that CS is caused by some abnormality in the immune system, similar to an allergy. Their common treatments are:

A. ALF:

Altered Lymphatic Factor (ALF) is a treatment that involves culturing a person's T-lymphocytes taken from their blood. The laboratory alters a portion of your blood through a complicated chemical process. This process supposedly allows the weaker cells to die and strengthens those remaining. Then a small amount of the altered blood is injected back into the individual in increasingly more concentrated doses to build up immunity and make the person more resistant to chemicals. As with some of these other esoteric treatments, they can only be done by specialists, tend to be expensive, and there is no hard data, only anecdotal reports as to their effectiveness.

B. Immune Boosters:

The list of items used is endless and includes everything from Enzyme Potentiated Desensitization (EPD), Vitamin C, Echinacea, Golden Seal, and other well known and esoteric ones from all over the world, as well as homeopathic remedies. The average success rate of these is less than 30%; yet 30% claim to have been helped. The danger is that many individuals are allergic or sensitive to them or become allergic or sensitive to these products, which for the most part are not regulated by the Food and Drug Administration.

Before one proceeds blindly on this course it is suggested that the substance be tested on yourself first, and periodically retested to make sure that you have not become sensitive to it. The way to do this is similar to the way described below; to test one's self for food sensitivities.

C. Provocation/Neutralization and Serial Dilution Testing:

These are procedures are designed to test various substances in order to ascertain if the patient is sensitive to them. They are also used to build up immunity to substances to which the patient reacts. The attempt to build up immunity is similar to immunological methods that have been used for years to treat biological allergies as well as some infectious diseases. In addition they are said to stop acute chemical, biological and food reactions. The exact mechanisms of how the later works are not fully understood

In a standard allergy practice the physician uses skin tests to determine sensitivity to a variety of knows allergens. A serum is then made up of the allergens that the individual reacted to and injected back into the patient periodically in doses of increasing concentrations. This stimulates the immune system to produce antibodies that make the person more resistant to those items they reacted to.

The environmental medical community argues that the above procedure is a one size fits all solution and is not applicable to individuals with chemical sensitivity. Therefore, they have altered the procedure so that it is specifically tailored to each individual and their sensitivities. Some expand the model beyond known biological allergens to chemicals and food.

Starting with a concentrated solution containing the suspected chemical, food, or chemical trigger, they inject .05 ml. just under the skin, and measure the subsequent wheel (bump) that develops. If the wheel either disappears or does not grow, and there are no physiological symptoms in an allotted time, (usually ten minutes) the assumption is that the individual is not sensitive to the injected substance.

If the individual is sensitive to this concentration, the size of the wheel will increase and/or they will experience systemic symptoms similar to those caused by a toxin. If this occurs within the allotted time, usually ten minutes, the person is deemed sensitive to that substance and the process is repeated with a less concentrated dilution. The process is repeated until the resultant wheel grows less than 2 cm. which is designated as the individual's end point. Then a serum of this strength is made and the individual instructed to use it twice daily, either by injection or sublingually to hopefully prevent (neutralize) additional reactions and build up immunity to the substance. Sometimes the patient is asked to report if the wheel grew at a later time to guard against delayed reactions.

Some practitioners test and determine the end points one at a time, others raise wheels. The later process is called Serial Dilution Testing.

Although the three surveys, Gibson, Johnson, and LeRoy, differ by a few some percentage points, they all agree that antigens that contain preservatives are more potentially harmful and less helpful than those without. Allison Johnson reports that for the preservative free group, 39% said that they were helped for inhalants, 37.5% for molds, 23% for foods, and 20% for chemicals. Ms. Johnson also notes that the treatment is much more effective on individuals whose end points do not change, and does not recommend it being used by individuals whose are constantly changing.[8] Obviously, end points have to be re-checked periodically.

While offering help, especially to individuals who are "allergic" to common biological allergens, versus sensitive to chemicals or the chemicals that molds produce, the treatment is expensive and time consuming. In order to be effective, testing has to be done by a very experienced tester in a safe environment that will not influence the results. In addition some physicians fear potential contamination of preservative free solutions, so it is very difficult to find physicians who are willing to use them and expose themselves to a possible lawsuit.

Food Allergies/Sensitivities:

Food sensitivities are often confused with food allergies. Even though the mechanisms are different, the symptoms are similar. Many PWCS develop sensitivities to various foods or the additives in the foods such as colorings and/or preservatives.

The most common causes of true food allergy are milk, eggs, peanuts, tree nuts, soybeans, wheat, crustaceans, and fish. Reactions can range from mild to severe. These can be tested for by skin or blood tests. The treatment is the same as for food sensitivities--avoidance. Some food allergies, especially those present at birth, are permanent and the foods should be avoided for life. Others, which develop later in life, tend to disappear if the food is avoided for a long enough time. At that point the food can be slowly added back into one's diet.

Some environmental physicians attempt to treat food sensitivities by Provocative Neutralization (PN) techniques. Others believe that food allergies, and even CS, are caused by an overgrowth of Candida Albicans, an intestinal yeast, a condition called Candidiasis, and treat food allergies by treating the patient for the yeast condition. [9]

Candidiasis is treated by a number of different methods depending on the severity of the yeast overgrowth and the philosophy of the health care

---

8. Johnson, "Survey Results from 351 Respondents," September 19, 1987, Brunswick, Maine

9. Numerous "popular" books have been written advocating this theory. For example see: William G. Crook, *The Yeast Connection: A Medical Breakthrough*, New York: Vintage, 1986. Yet, too often, health care professionals will automatically assume and treat yeast and parasites without obtaining laboratory confirmation. Needless to say, the only thing that improves with this approach is the bank account of the physician.

professional. Mild cases are treated by diet, specifically a low to zero carbohydrate diet, in an attempt to starve the yeast because the yeast thrives on sugar. Other practitioners use various natural and synthetic substances that range from herbs, garlic, and colloidal silver, to prescription anti-fungal drugs such as Nystatin, and PN techniques.

Very often the patient gets worse during treatment. CS physicians call this phenomena "die off" or a Herxheimer reaction.[10] The Herxheimer reaction is caused by substances released by the dying yeast cells, and if it occurs, should cease in two or three days. Others use PN as an attempt to build up immunity to yeast. These and other such methods to treat Candidiasis and food sensitivities should only be attempted after ascertaining that there truly is an overgrowth of yeast in the intestinal track and a careful analysis of the risk to reward ratio found in the appendix of this book.

CS specialist physicians believe that Candidiasis is a real, documented medical condition. They also note that many of their chemically sensitive patients have an overgrowth of yeast. But they do not believe that yeast is the primary cause of CS. They believe it is a secondary problem resulting from the primary cause, chemical poisoning which has altered the intestinal track. They argue that by addressing the secondary, rather than the primary cause, the physicians are not getting at the root of the problem, chemical toxicity from broken detoxification system which leads to neural sensitization.

They have found that as an individual gets their chemical exposure under control, yeast and food related problems tend to lessen. They will obviously treat a yeast infection if it has been documented by a reputable laboratory test.

The most effective, least expensive, most harmless and widely used method to treat food sensitivities by most informed health professionals is to avoid foods that cause reactions, and eating as much organic and natural food as possible to eliminate ingesting chemicals and additives which could cause problems.

To lessen the chances of the PWCS developing reactions to foods, they also advocate a food rotation diet. The most common one is to eat a food that can be tolerated once every four days. If the commonly available foods are causing problems, and one does not have enough of them to rotate, there are many sources to obtain exotic foods such as venison, boar, etc.

Rotation diets have proven successful for about 75% of those surveyed

---

10.www.whatcausesyeastinfections.org/candida-die-off/

in the published surveys. Further indications that the food sensitivity problem is caused by a chemical overload are the reports from individuals who have achieved a chemically free-living lifestyle and environment. Many report that after they lived there for a while, their food sensitivities have lessened or disappeared entirely without specific treatment for food sensitivities.

Paying attention to food sensitivities and getting them under control is obviously important, because if CS progresses the individual may find themselves without any tolerated foods to eat, and in extreme cases, a feeding tube may have to be inserted.

Many environmental physicians recommend treating acute food reactions by: taking an antacid such as half a teaspoonful of Tri-Salts or Alka-Seltzer Gold™ to create a alkaline rather than acidic environment; Milk of Magnesia to clear the "gut;" and by administering a .1 cc "neutralizing" dose of histamine, the proper dose of which would have been routinely obtained during PN testing by an environmental physician. No one is quite sure how this homeopathic intervention works, but it is not harmful and many individuals report success.

If an acute reaction occurs while being tested, the physician will often administer a high dose IV of Vitamin C and inhaled oxygen. Many individuals report that this later intervention stopped the reaction.

Robert S. Mayer Ph.D.

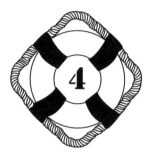

Your Home

The best strategy to combat and manage CS is to live in a safe, nontoxic house located in an area that has clean, or more realistically, "good enough" air. This of course is easier said than done. Impulsively moving in the hope of finding an area of the country where one will feel better is not advised until all other options to maintain yourself in your present environment have been exhausted.

Pollution free air is becoming more and more difficult, if not impossible to find in the United States. Unfortunately, at present, there is no central agency to which one can turn for advice or analysis of different possible areas. PWCS greatly need safe housing communities, or hospitals to which one can run, if in trouble, but these are not available. All areas of the country contain potential known and unknown problems and therefore require a trade of one toxin for another.

Difficult choices have to be made. The choice that one makes is individual and must be carefully thought through. What works for one might not work for another. Leaving a geographic location that one is used to where one's friends and relatives live is usually difficult, even for healthy people, and many people who have done so eventually return home. They do so even if their original home is more toxic than the area to which they moved. The reasons are usually loneliness, and/or discomfort with the new unfamiliar environment.

Other individuals moved to a "safe" place, hoping that if they stay there long enough they will be healthy enough to return home to their previous life. Many have found that they cannot achieve this goal. Living in a clean area for a length of time one feels better because the system is not being assaulted by chemicals. The masking that the body did that allowed the PWCS to marginally exist in their old toxic place wears off in the new place. But since the real problem, chemical toxicity from a broken detoxification system has not been fixed, when the unmasked PWCS attempts to triumphantly return to their previous environment, often they find it even more intolerable than before they left.

Therefore, running to hopeful safety, even though that is what your terrified survival instincts are telling you to do, is not the first choice. Moving to another place should only be attempted after all efforts to clean up the current environment or finding a better microclimate in you home territory have been exhausted and there is no other choice. Needless to stay it is definitely not advised to remain in an environment that cannot be made "good enough." Un-arrested CS is a progressive neurological disease. The end point of this progression could be increased sensitivity to a myriad of substances and possible damage to vital organs.

The following chapters will discuss how to make your home and its immediate environment safer. In many cases it is possible to save the house and make it good enough for tolerable living and possible healing. This chapter will relate what the readership of *Our Toxic Times* have done, and the products they found helpful to eliminate toxic items from the home, substituting them with products that are tolerable for them. In addition it will present some ideas on how to make the house generally safer.

General Ideas For Your Home [1]

Do whatever possible in the house to reduce the number of items that could be offgassing symptom producing, brain damaging toxins. The task is large and appears overwhelming. The illness has probably depleted your energy, and your support network has most likely gotten smaller. However, you must do the best you can to eliminate any known or possible toxin from your immediate, controllable environment.

- If in doubt, throw it out. Less is more.

- Clean and de-clutter your home. Less "stuff" equates to less chances of the "stuff" offgassing toxins, which might enter your system. If you have problems simplifying try looking at the *Simplify Your Life Books* by Elaine St. James.[2]

- If you aren't sure what is bothering you and don't know where to start, the most likely suspects will be found in your food, home, work place, personal care products, clothing, cleaning products, and electronic equipment, all of which are probably loaded with various chemicals.

- You can substitute safe products for the ones that you are accustomed to.[3]

- Do not store items for possible future use in a public storage facility as they have, more likely than not, been treated with a pesticide or cleaned with a substance that will get into the "precious" stored items and they will become contaminated.

- Clean galvanized garbage cans with lids are perfect for storing many items, as are tolerated plastic boxes, which can be kept in a separate area of the house such as a garage.

- Health comes before sentiment.

---

1. The following information comes from members of the Chemical Injury Information Network (CIIN). Additional information can be found in any of the numerous books have been written on how to fix and build a safe home. See: *Healthy House and Healthy House Building* by John Bower; *Healthy House Answer Book*, by John and Lynn Marie Bower; *Healthy by Design*, by Rousseau and Wesley; *Your Home, Your Health, & Well-Being*, by David Rousseau, W.J. Rea, M.D. and Jean Enwright, or your local support group can probably refer you to a local expert.

2. See books by Elaine St James. She has written a number of them, which can be obtained from www.amazon.com.

3. This will be discussed in future chapters.

- The things you remove can always be stored and tested later for safety. If they are found safe, they can be added back.

- Questionable objects can be covered with foil, barrier cloth or medical grade Tyvek™. After covering, observe after a while if the room smells better, or more importantly if you feel better, since every thing that "smells" does not necessarily get you sick.[4]

- At best, the house should not have any carpeting, new or untested furniture, plants, fountains, or anything that will support mold growth, soft plastic, vinyl, fragrances, candles, potpourri, plug-ins, air fresheners, toxic cleaning products, toilet bowel cleansers, pesticides, moth balls, herbicides or fertilizers.

- If the house has "hung" ceilings, replace the standard most likely porous sections, which will absorb odors, moisture and support mold, with metal or some other nonporous, nontoxic product.

- Any of the "safe" low VOC paints are a good sealant for wallboard. Choose which brand by testing samples to determine your individual sensitivities.

- Test proposed paint by painting a small piece of metal such as baked aluminum, let it thoroughly dry and cure. Place the cured sample in a covered mason jar for a while. Then cautiously smell and note if you have any symptoms. If in doubt, and want to be sure, sleep with the sample near you.

- Oil-based paint is best to seal walls. However, this is a tricky solution, as oil paint needs about six months or more to fully offgass. Very sensitive people that do not have a milk allergy have used Milk Paint successfully, however, it is not a good sealer for the walls.

- Unpainted plaster walls also work well if one can find a craftsman to do the work.

- Change gas/propane hot water heaters to electric hot water heaters that will automatically make hot water when needed. (On demand).

---

4. Medical grade Tyvek can be purchased from Dupont: 856-952-3300 or Taylor Designs: 802-365-4840. Barrier cloth can be purchased from any place that sells cotton goods for the chemically sensitive such as Janice's, 1-800-526-4237, www.janices.com.

- If possible move the furnace outside and down wind of the house, or vent it to the outside.

- The house should not have any gas/propane appliances.

- If the gas/propane stove cannot be removed, turn off the gas/propane supply. Cook on a hot plate, and/or toaster oven.

- Gas fired forced air heat is very toxic.

- Electric baseboard heat is good if not electrically sensitive, but expensive.

- If you can afford it, convert to baseboard hot water heat.

- Do not use microwave ovens. Some professionals claim that they change the molecular consistency of the food, and are very bad if you have EMF sensitivity.

- Existing ductwork should be inspected for dirt and mold. They can be cleaned, using a commercial duct cleaning service that will agree to use new or clean brushes with a solution of hydrogen peroxide or trisodium phosphate (TSP).

- Throw away your toxic furniture polishes. Wood furniture can easily be cleaned with a mixture of olive oil and lemon juice, and beeswax.[5]

- Many people do not like to polish furniture as the polish can collect dust. They prefer to clean and dust with a damp cloth.

- Metal lawn type furniture and glass tables are the safest furniture.[6]

- If necessary, have 100% cotton cushions made for the metal furniture.

- Wash off all new metal products such as furniture, duct work, etc. with a solution of Tri Sodium Phosphate (TSP) before bringing them into the house as the manufacturing process leaves an oil film on them.[7]

---

5. Bemis Manufacturing Co. 1-800-558-7651 makes a good wood conditioner for cutting boards, wood blocks, and knives that is free from taste or odor.

6. There are firms advertising in Our Toxic Times that claim to make nontoxic furniture. Neither I, nor responders to the surveys have had any personal experience with them. They will, however, ship you samples of their materials free of charge for you to test them.

7. TSP needs to be activated in hot water. Although not very corrosive, gloves and eye protection should be used.

- Give all new items time to air out, preferably in the sun before bringing them into your home.

- To remove pesticide residue from molding, etc. use TSP followed by a solution of baking soda in water.

- New heating, ventilating and air conditioning (HVAC) filters often have a smell when they are unwrapped. If the smell bothers you, leave new filters exposed to the air, preferably in the sun, until the smell is reduced.

- Many filters are made with glues, synthetics and other toxic substances. They may or may not bother you. Test before use.

- Keep a supply of offgassed air and heating filters in the house, in the event that the one in use gets contaminated.

- Inspect filters monthly, and change them when both sides get gray in order to maintain the purity of the household air and protect the HVAC coils and duct work from accumulating dirt.

- Learn to read product labels as carefully as you do food and supplement labels.

- Get Manufacturer's Product Safety Data Sheets (MSDS) for any product you are considering using to learn about the ingredients it contains and the toxicity of the ingredients.

- Find or construct a way to enter the house indirectly such as through a garage or mudroom. This will enable you to leave the clothes you wore out in other environments, thus reducing the toxins entering your house. If this chamber has a bathroom and/or changing room, so much the better. This "chamber" will obviously help reduce the amount of outside toxins that enter your home even more so.

- Don't wear your shoes into the house, as they will carry contaminants in. Keep safe slippers for your guests.

- Weather-strip outside doors and put a non-rubber sweep on the bottom to reduce the toxins that might enter.

- Offgas the sweep, if necessary, before you install it.

- Or install a sill for the door to close on.

- Use old fashioned felt weather-striping, or white foam, rather than high-tech ones containing rubber or an unknown material.

- Test it first, and if necessary air it out before use.

- Seal the joints all over the house where the outside wall and floor meet with a safe sealant to prevent outside air infiltration.[8]

- Seal as many openings and places in the house that will allow outside air to enter, as possible. For sealing jobs use 100% silicon if you can tolerate it. The silicone product with the least amount of other ingredients in it, although not perfect, tends to be best.

- Silicone will cure and become nontoxic given enough time. The smell is strong at first.

- To cure it faster, use a hair dryer, and cover it with paper masking tape. It will cure even though covered. When cured, tape removes easily.

- Silicone formulas are constantly changing, so self-test before use and avoid any product containing a fungicide, pesticide, or algaecides. If in doubt, contact the company.[9]

- Metal tape is very good to seal and/or cover up various things.[10]

- A temporary cheap solution is to cover suspicious areas with aluminum foil, shiny side out, and metal tape, or Tu-Tuf.[11]

- Great Stuff™ is also an excellent sealant. It has a short lived toxic smell as it is sprayed out of the aerosol can and should be done by someone who is not sensitive. It is nontoxic after it dries.[12]

---

8. Commonly used sealants are silicone, metal tape and Great Stuff™.

9. Respondents have reported success with OSI, VP 275 Silicone™. OSI Sealants, Inc., Henkel Consumer Adhesives, Professional Division, Mentor, Ohio 44060.

10. Many metal tapes have a toxic smell. The best is Shurtape, at the time of this writing, which can be obtained from E.L. Faust & Co. Caution and discussion with them is advised as the formula is constantly changing. E.L. Faust will send a sample for personal testing.

11. Tu-tuf™ can be obtained at numerous building supply places such as Sto-Cote Products, 800-535-2621, or Nirvana Safe Haven, 800-868-9355.

12. Great Stuff™ is readily available at sources such as The Home Depot and Lowe's. It expands as it is applies, and a little goes a long way. Excess can be removed wet, or cut with a razor blade when dry.

- Avoid any sealer that has a mold retardants in it.

- Seal any wood that has an odor that you react to. There are numerous products on the market that claim to seal in toxins, but many individuals cannot tolerate them. Success has been reported with old fashioned shellac.

- Shellac is very toxic when applied, but the smell quickly dissipates.

- Any particleboard or chipboard doors, shelves, etc. should be removed and discarded if they cannot be completely covered or sealed.

- Less toxic alternative materials for cabinets are: metal, glass, and offgassed hardwoods that have been thoroughly sealed.

- Although everyone is different, many people find poplar non-toxic.

- If you can find it, kiln dried poplar is very best.

- Some PWCS have trouble purchasing items from large chain type stores such as The Home Depot or Lowes, as they sell many toxic products including pesticides. The pollutants from these products might bother you when you shop, or be on the product that you purchase and thus, into your home. If you fall into that category, it is best to purchase online or from a smaller specialty store.

- If the outside air becomes toxic from a fire, wood smoke, etc., try using metal tape on all possible cracks in the house, windows and doors to help block fumes.

- Be sure to have some way to get clean fresh air, or air the house out periodically as PWCS must have fresh air coming in a good part of the time as everything has a smell.

- It the outside air is toxic most of the time, you need to seriously consider moving.

- Air rises in a multi-level building, so be careful of what is below you, such as a below ground parking garage, smoking neighbors or a moldy basement.

- Cover, or remove your window air conditioner in the winter to reduce drafts and keep out wood smoke or other toxins.

- Control the humidity in the house. A house with relative humidity under 50% is less likely to grow mold and support dusts mites.

- If you choose a commercial dehumidifier, only use one that has a metal case, and inspect it regularly for possible mold buildup.[13]

- The best place for a dehumidifier is on the lowest level of the house, such as the basement. This will also reduce the noise.

- Arrange to have the dehumidifier empty outside of the house or into a slop sink, not into the pail that comes with it, This will make your life easier and lessen the chance of mold build up.

- Increasing airflow by using fans will help control mold.

- Give mold as little to grow on as possible by reducing soft goods.

- Run a fan in the basement, and laundry room to keep the air moving, to prevent mold.

- Run the fan on your HVAC system 24/7 to keep the coils and duct work dry to prevent mold buildup and filter particles from the house.

- Do not use any machine or filtration device that uses or emits ozone. Even though ozone is an excellent odor remover, it is very toxic to breathe and does not dissipate as fast as the manufacturers claim.

- If you must use ozone, have a professional apply it when you and your pets are not in the house.

- When the treatment is finished, have the service run kitchen and bathroom exhaust fans to get the ozone out.

- Multiply by ten the ozone machine manufacturer's recommended time to re-enter the house.

- Re-enter cautiously, as ozone damages lung tissue. You should not be able to smell it.

- Turn the air in the house over as much as possible with clean HEPA filtered air, through a Heat Recovery Ventilator ducted to remove stale

---

13. Sears sells a metal dehumidifier. Larger more powerful ones, with a HEPA filter, can be purchased from Thermastore, 800-533-7533, www.thermastor.com.

air from bathrooms and closets.

- Unplug all other electric appliances in the house when not in use. The computer devices placed in them to maintain the settings keep the wires warm, and thus the supposedly "off" electronic device continues to emit low level toxic fumes.

- Remove outlet and switch plate covers and spray in Great Stuff™ as the channels that the wires run in go all the way to the basement, which may contain toxins. As mentioned before, air always rises in a building.

- Specially made sealing plates are also available at electrical supply stores.

- Purchase baby proof outlet covers and plug them in to any unused outlets in the house. This is another way to close off channels that might bring contaminated air into the house from inside the walls and lower levels.

- An electrician can remove the box, seal up all the cracks, replace it and thus it will be sealed.

- Leave the door to your washing machine open when not in use to discourage mold growth in the machine.

- Put some baking soda in the washing machine when not in use to absorb odors and prevent mold build up from any remaining water.

- Never leave wet clothes in the machine for any length of time. Best to remove and dry them as quickly as possible.

- Create a test space in your home: Find an enclosed space that is clean and empty. To test an object, simply place it in the test room. Close the door and any HVAC vent in the room. Leave the item there for a few hours or a day, then gently stick your nose in and cautiously smell. Note what happens to you. The room can also be used to offgass new items.

Other Suggestions

- Keep a covered metal garbage can next to the mailbox to throw away junk mail and any mail that contains fragrance.

- Ask to be taken off any mailing lists that use scented products.

- Write to Mail Preference Service to get your name taken off junk mail/3rd class mail lists to reduce the amount of paper in the house.[14]

- Magazines, if a problem, can be left flipped open in a garage, put under your windshield wiper or the trunk of your car until offgassed. For extreme cases, rip out and separate the pages and hang on a clothesline in the sun until they are tolerable.

- When placing orders from a store or a catalogue, request that no scented items be placed in the order.

- Do everything you can to prevent oil or gas fumes from entering the house.

- Bathrooms, laundry rooms, and other such areas should be fitted with exhaust fans venting outside.

- Seal the basement and any inside the house garage from the rest of the house, with airtight doors and recommended safe sealant.

- Keep the basement and garage under negative pressure with exhaust fans to prevent the stale and possibly contaminated air from flowing into the living space.

- Keep the rest of the house under slight positive pressure to prevent toxins from leaching from the walls. This can be done with an intake fan attached to a HEPA air filter.

- Do not store or start vehicles or lawn maintenance motors in an attached or below the home garage.

---

14. Mail Preference Service, P.O. Box 282, Carmel, NY 10512. There is a one dollar fee, the form can be downloaded at www.dmaconsumers.org/mailform.php

Removing Odors from the Outside of Electronics[15]

- Most outside cases or coverings of electronic equipment have oil or some other coating from the manufacturing process. To remove it, use Everclear™ or grain alcohol from a liquor store. If you are sensitive to these, do it outside. Wipe the telephone, keyboard etc. It dries quickly and doesn't ruin the electronics.

- If you are sensitive to VOC emissions from a television set or other electronic item, encase it in a vented box, which can be built out of safe, sealed wood, metal or glass. If possible, put an exhaust fan and dryer vent hose on the case to take the fumes to an air cleaner or out of the living space.

- If you are sensitive to VOC or EMF emission from computers, put the tower in a vented box or in another room and run long cables to the keyboard, monitor and mouse. The monitor should be well outgassed.

- Another option to increase the distance between you and the computer or laptop, is with a wireless keyboard and mouse.

- If necessary, increase the font size to make reading easier from a distance.

- Some people tolerate laptops better than desk computers, others do not.

- PWCS find used or store display models that have had time to offgass more tolerable, unless they have been saturated with fragrance.

- A small fan blowing the fumes away, work for many.

- People seem to have more success with plasma monitors.

- Others have had success by placing a piece of glass two or three inches in front of the monitor.

- Run new items somewhere away from you for as long as it take the item to offgass.

---

15. When electronic equipment runs, wires and other parts heat up causing toxic VOCs to enter the environment. Often equipment that is older and has been run for a while does not have this problem.

Electromagnetic Sensitivity

- The best way to feel better is to move away from the EMF source.

- Purchase a hand held EMF meter to take readings at locations in your home to find problem areas, to avoid them or to eliminate them.

- Have an expert assess your house for wiring problems, some can be corrected to reduce the EMFs.

- Individuals who are EMF sensitive react badly to dimmer switches and therefore they should be removed from the house of these individuals.

- If EMF sensitive, use as many battery appliances as possible.

- If you are EMF sensitive use a battery powered or wind up clock.

- Avoid florescent lights; the flicker gives some PWCS symptoms.

- Incandescent lights, although less energy efficient are better tolerated for people with EMS than fluorescents.

- If having a symptom, try grounding yourself in salt water or walking on the ground with bare feet.

- When using a computer or any other electrical appliance don't wear rubber sneakers or rubber sole shoes. Being barefoot is best as it will help you stay grounded.

- Metal beds and furniture tend to act like antennas and attract EMF.

- Turn off electricity in the bedroom at the source, (circuit breaker or fuse box) so that your body will not be exposed while you sleep.

- If necessary, a relay switch can be installed in the bedroom that will turn the electricity off at the circuit breaker or fuse box.

- Have an electrician inspect your home to make sure that it is properly grounded.

The Immediate Area Outside of the House

- If possible remove all trees and shrubs that shade the house to allow the sun to dry the house and thus prevent any mold or mildew growth.

- Asphalt driveways or walks should be avoided if possible, as they emit toxins when the sun shines on them.

- Especially avoid fresh asphalt.

- Cement, paving blocks, or even gravel are better.

- Give up on the idea of having a perfect lawn. Just cut whatever grows short, removing the cuttings so they will not "rot" if left on the grass. If you must weed, do it by hand.

- Sod is usually grown with herbicides and should be avoided. It also has to be watered and fertilized regularly to maintain its "golf course like" appearance.

- Convert your expensive to maintain, fertilize and pesticide devouring lawn to an organic garden. You will then be sure that the food you grow and eat will really be organic and not exposed to toxins picked up from the farm to the store, or sprayed with something to make it more appealing.[16]

- Weeds in the cracks of the cement walk can be burned off with a torch when you are not present, killed with nontoxic weed killer products, salt water and vinegar, or removed by hand.

- Organic gardening is an excellent hobby that gets you in fresh air, gives you good food to eat, and the exercise is a fringe benefit.

- Strawberries work well in some areas and provide excellent ground cover as well as a treat.

---

16. The only problem with this is that neighborhood dogs will gravitate to your pesticide free lawn because they are smarter than people. If you do not want the free fertilizer, there are innumerable sound emitting devices on the market to keep them and rodents away. Spreading human urine around also works as they will stay away from a territory "marked" by a larger animal.

General Items to Avoid

This is a general list, obviously some people can tolerate more than others:

- Rubber.

- Polyvinylchloride (PVC).

- Vinyl.

- Soft plastic, (many people can tolerate hard plastics and Formica ™).

- Chip board

- Latex

- Sealers that do not harden and become odor free.

- Any new item that has an odor that gives you symptoms.

- Cements, adhesives,(Elmer's Glue™ is reported to be safe).

- Fresh paint.

- All fossil fuels.

- Electronic air filters.

- Newsprint.

- Rubbing alcohol.

- Refrigerants.

- Spray containers.

- Insecticides.

- Plastic air conditioning and heating ducts.

- Moth balls.

- Ammonia.

- Clorox.

- Brass, silver, and shoe polish.

- Pine Christmas trees, (some people tolerate holly).

- Candles, especially scented, (beeswax works for some).

- Anything else that is highly scented.

- Oil lamps, fire places, gas or wood smoke.

- Propane. If you must use it, be sure to be upwind of the flame and tank.

- Dark colored items. In general, light colored items are usually safer than dark colored ones because of the dyes used. This includes wall colors, clothing, and furniture.

- Prescription antidepressant medication, as the surveys show that most people get sick from them.

- Coated pills and tablets.

- Colored liquid medication.

- Medication in capsule form is generally better than tablets.

- If the capsule is a problem, the mediation can be emptied out and taken directly or mixed with water or juice, or put in a clear gelatin capsule.

- Steroids—avoid unless absolutely medically necessary.

- The doctors will erroneous tell you that steroids nasally/orally inhaled, or topically applied are not absorbed. They are wrong. They are systemically absorbed. Use only in an emergency.

- Any food that contains colors, dyes, preservatives, artificial flavors, and ingredients especially the ones that you cannot pronounce. Organic food is best, and is recommended.

- Just because the label says it is "natural" does not make it safe. Arsenic is a natural product, as is organic tobacco.

- Moldy foods. Frozen fruit tends to reduce the possibility of mold, as the food is flash-frozen right after it is picked.

- Food treatments and contaminants. Soak or wash fresh fruit in a solution of hydrogen peroxide to remove toxins from the outer layer, such as fertilizers, pesticides, and anything else they may have picked up in their journey from the ground to you.

- Most foods that comes in a can or cardboard box.

- Food cooked on an open flame. The food will absorb the odor of the cooking fuel. Electric is the safest way to cook.

- Aluminum cooking utensils. Corning makes a fine line of glass pots and pans. They are hard to find, but often are on Ebay.com.

- Printers, fax machines, and copy machines, especially when running.

- Newly constructed or recently remodeled places.

- Any machine that emits ozone.

Robert S. Mayer Ph.D.

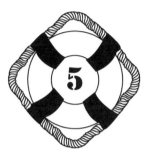

The Bedroom

A nontoxic, safe bedroom sanctuary is essential to regain as much of your health as possible. In such an oasis, where the average person spends eight hours, the body will have a chance to eliminate stored toxins, detoxify, and regain health. It can also be used as a safe place to run to, in case another part of the house becomes toxic for one reason or another.

Your tolerance to various substances will probably increase as you clean up your house and sleep in a nontoxic bedroom. Thus the range of products that can be used, the odors you can tolerate, the activities you can do, and places you can go will increase.[1]

The following are strategies the readership of Our Toxic Times used to make a bedroom as toxin free as possible.[2]

---

1. In some cases, individuals feel worse at first. Living in a toxin free environment encourages the release of stored toxins in the body which, until removed, might make one feel sick again. The problem is time limited.

2. Even though the contributors have found the following products "safe", obviously everyone is different and it is prudent to test a product before you use it. If you find one to be safe for you, it is wise to stockpile a supply as formulas often change without notice.

The Bedroom Oasis

- Remove everything from the bedroom except a nontoxic bed and bedding.

- Well offgassed hardwood floors work for many people.

- Ceramic tile floors are safest.

- If the bedroom is carpeted, remove it and unless you find hard wood flooring beneath it, cover the sub flooring with ceramic tiles.

- If you cannot do this, cover the carpet or floor with heavy gage aluminum foil, medical grade Tyvek, and/or barrier cloth.[3]

- Do not cover a concrete floor with foil or other materials that block airflow, as this will inhibit moisture circulation and mold will grow under the foil.

- Remove all curtains, drapes, shades, or other hangings, from the windows and replace them with metal or well offgassed wooden blinds.

- Vertical blinds are best as vertical surfaces collect less dust than horizontal ones.

- Remove all clothes from any closet that opens directly to the room and seal the door to hold in any old residues of dry cleaning etc.

- If needed, install an exhaust in this closet that can empty the air outside the house.

- If possible, build or create another closet in another place in the house and seal off the original closet door with metal tape to hold in any old residues of dry cleaning etc.[4]

- Remove all electronic equipment and appliances from the bedroom except a metal air cleaner.

---

3. Barrier cloth can be purchased from any place that sells cotton goods for the chemically sensitive such as Janice's, 1-800-526-4237, www.janices.com.

4. The least toxic metal tape used to be Polyken™, which can be obtained from E.L. Fousts Co., Inc 1-800-353-6878, www.foustco.com., however Tyco the manufacturer of this tape has recently changed its formula and the new one is causing reactions in some people. Foust is recommending Shurtape AF973, the safety of which this author does not have any information on. Check with Foust before ordering, they will make suggestions and send you samples.

- If electromagnetically sensitive, use a battery operated, or wind up clock to lessen electrical wire odors and prevent sensitivity problems.

Beds

- A safe bed for the extremely sensitive individual can be made by covering a ceramic or hardwood floor with a number of layers of thick, best quality possible, white, well washed, cotton towels. On a hard surface, the towels make a tolerable mattress.[5]

- Wash the towels often in baking soda and hot water to keep odors and the dust mite population down.

- Many PWCS are able to tolerate a cotton futon on the floor or on a metal or well offgassed frame.

- Cover the futon with a removable, washable cotton cover made of barrier cloth to protect you from manufacturing residue and reduce the possibility of dust mites.

- If necessary wrap the futon it with a layer of medical grade Tyvek™ or Tu-Tuff™ before covering it with barrier cloth.

- A metal bed frame or a metal army cot with a well washed, 100% cotton mattress pad for a mattress, although not the most comfortable, works well as a nontoxic bed and was used in the Environmental Unit in TriCity Hospital, Dallas, TX when it was operational.[6]

- Bed frames should be made of well offgassed hard wood, such as poplar, maple or metal.

- If the finish on wooden bed frames is a problem, one or two coats of shellac are an excellent nontoxic sealer for many.

- Many use 100% cotton futons, covered with a washable barrier cloth cover successfully.

- An older mattress can work if you have covered with either heavy gauge

---

5. Large, white, 100% cotton towels have many uses for the extremely sensitive. They can be used to cover any surface that you sleep or sit on thus offering protection.

6. Humans are like weeds, we get used to almost anything.

aluminum foil, Tu-Tuff™, medical grade Tyvek™, and/or barrier cloth.[7]

- You can obtain new mattresses without flame retardants with a doctor's prescription from most mattress manufacturers.

- There are also numerous local firms that will custom make a mattress for you. They can be found in the local yellow pages or on line.

- Organic cotton mattresses are available and many readers report success, but others report that they "smell" worse than the one that was replaced. As always, test any mattress before you purchase it, as they are expensive, especially the organic ones.

Sheets:

- For most respondents, neutral or white, well-laundered, high thread count sheets from the best manufacturers work well. Some readers prefer organic. As noted above, many claim that organic cotton smells worse than regular sheets, and they react to them. You will have to decide which works best.

Pillows:

- For the extremely sensitive, use a folded white cotton towel that can be washed at least weekly to remove dust mites, and body smells. The towel can be covered with a "safe" 100 per cent cotton pillowcase" if the roughness of the towel bothers you.

- For the less sensitive, an older cotton pillow that has been covered with medical grade Tyvek™, barrier cloth, and a quality, high thread count pillowcase might work.

- Some PWCS can even tolerate feather pillows and blends. As always, test first.

- Some people can tolerate "hypo-allergenic" pillows, or pillows filled with wool, and even synthetic blends. Again, test before you buy. [8]

---

7. Tu-Tuff can be obtained at most building supply places such as Shelter Supply, 1-800-762-8399.

8. Most advertised hypoallergenic pillowcases and mattress covers are made from plastic or synthetic material and should be avoided.

Blankets:

- For the very sensitive, use well-washed, large, white cotton towels work well as a blanket.

- Wash blankets often in baking soda or just very hot water to remove dust mites.

- Cotton blankets can be layered for added warmth.

- Some people are able to tolerate wool blankets.

- 100% cotton comforters or quilts usually work well. Again, wash often to control dust mites.

- If the blanket of choice cannot be washed, e.g. wool, or a comforter which cannot fit into the washing machine, cover them with a removable barrier cloth cover that can be washed.

- Use a top sheet; with a very high thread count, made of 100% cotton between you and the blanket, which can be washed frequently.

- For added safety, place another sheet on top of the blanket. This system can be washed more frequently and easier than blankets or quilts, which are hard to fit in most washing machines, and thus give you added protection from dust mites.

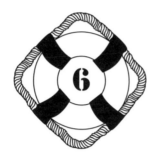

The Rest of the House

Drinking Water Supply

- Municipal water is not advisable as it contains chlorine as a disinfectant, and perhaps other ingredients as well as the possibility of pesticides from lawns leaching into the water supply.

- Bottled or filtered water is the common solution.

- You may have to try a number of bottled waters to find one that agrees with you.

- Batches from the same water company can vary.

- Note the batch number of water that suddenly disagrees with you. If it is bottled, it may be the time of the year that the equipment used to filter and/or bottle the water was subjected to a vigorous cleaning.

- Distilled water that you distill at home is safest however, you must take mineral supplements with it or you will get sick.[1]

---

1. It is better to distill it yourself, as commercially available distilled water comes in soft plastic containers, which leach polymers into the water. Soft plastic bottles are can absorb the odors of items they were stored next to.

- You can make your own purified water by installing a reverse osmosis water filtration unit, preferably one made out of stainless steel.

- Water in plastic containers is not advised as the plastic leaches into the water and as soft plastic containers are porous, they might pick up pollutants from the store.

- The majority of the respondents prefer glass bottled water.

- Mountain Valley Spring Water comes in glass containers.[2]

- A ceramic water filtering unit can be installed on the sink or free standing.

- Well water must be periodically tested for contaminants.

- To filter household water, install a two-part whole house water filter on the incoming water supply to remove chlorine, fluoride, and general impurities. Your skin, the largest organ in the body, can absorb common toxins found in city water such as: chlorine, fluoride, pesticides and fertilizers from lawn runoff, or any other number of contaminants.

- If the above is not practical, a carbon filter that you simply screw onto the showerhead or sink faucet can be purchased at Home Depot, Lowe's, or other such sources. They are not recommended for drinking water, but will remove most if the above additives.

Appliances

- The washing machine should have a ceramic or stainless steel drum and inside material.

- The same rule applies to the dishwasher.

- In purchasing a new dishwasher, beware of any insulated with observable black tar like material, as they almost never offgass.

- Less expensive dishwashers have fiberglass insulation. They are generally be nosier, but less toxic.

- To clean a new machine, run a few empty loads with TSP and baking soda.

---

2. www.mountainvalleyspring.com.

- If it is a machine that scented products have been used in, try multiple washes with TSP and baking soda. Sometimes it works. If not, discard the machine.

- Leave the washer door open when not in use to lessen mold build up.

- Put some baking soda in a machine that is not in use for the same reason, as some water may remain in the bottom of the machine.

- Have the laundry room as far away from the bedroom and general living area as possible.

- Basements or garages are the best place for the laundry area.

- If the laundry room must be in the living area, and you have central air conditioning, and /or forced air heat, cut off the air ducts to that area to prevent the odors and moisture from traveling to the rest of the house.

- Fit the laundry room with an exhaust fan.

- Run the fan 24/7, in the laundry room to keep the air circulating and prevent mold growth, as the humidity tends to be high in this area.

Books and Other Reading Material

- Reading might be difficult for the chemically sensitive because of the possible toxicity of the paper and/or ink.

- Some papers, books, and ink are better than others.

- Material printed on shiny paper is the worst, and best avoided.

- Books from lending libraries may be a problem. Many have picked up the odors of individuals who have borrowed them before. Smell first.

- Reading boxes can be purchased or constructed. They are enclosed boxes with a glass top and holes to put in your hands, keeping the odors from the item away from the PWCS. Or, try placing a glass plate or a cellophane reading bag over the material to be read and if necessary, turn the pages with the eraser end of a pencil.

- Purchase books new so they can be returned if you can't tolerate them.

- Most books will offgass if let alone for a while.

- Listening to books on tape or CD is a good solution for the very sensitive.

- Any perfume from previous listeners that is troublesome can be removed from the cassette with grain alcohol.

- Books that smell might be made readable if baked in an oven for 35 minutes at 250F.

- One respondent stores books and odorous items in the trunk of her car, when weather is warm, for a few weeks before she attempts to read them.

- To safely store books in the home, place them in zip lock bags, or in bookcases behind glass doors.

- The bookcase can be vented outside, using a small computer fan purchased at Radio Shack or some other supplier, connected to metal duct work, through a sealed hole in the wall, or under a double hung window.

Office Supplies and Computers

- If you cannot use a computer or electric typewriter, try a manual. However, the ink on the ribbon or lubrication may be a problem.

- If you are very sensitive, use highest cotton (rag) content paper for writing. It is less toxic than paper made from wood fiber and it will possibly be less harsh to the touch.

- Soy based ink is nontoxic for most.

- If Scotch Tape™ bothers you; test various house brands.

- Carbonless paper is very toxic and should be avoided.

- A computer is of great benefit. If tolerated, become computer literate.

- You can learn this skill at home with tutorials. An added benefit is that learning new skills keeps the brain sharp.

- Older computers are better for PWCS than newer ones.

- Used computers are also a good option. They are outgassed, cheaper and in good supply from any local computer repair shop.

- Word of caution: be careful with used, as they may have lingering perfume smells from previous owner. As always, test with your nose.

- Another option is to purchase a new one, run it constantly in another room until the manufacturing smells are gone.

- Do not buy used equipment without smelling it first, e.g. never buy such equipment online as you cannot smell test for tolerance.

- LCD (liquid crystal display) monitors emit fewer toxins than CRT (cathode ray tube) ones.

- If the computer still bothers you, move the "brain" of the computer to another location with an extension cord and if necessary, a cordless keyboard and mouse.

- You can also place a reading box over the monitor with a small fan drawing the fumes to another area.

- If the fan alone doesn't solve the problem, vent the reading box outside.

- A simple household fan might also work to blow any possible smells from the computer away from you.

- If necessary, cover the keyboard with cellophane or try saran wrap.

- Some people prefer laptops. Others cannot tolerate them for various reasons and can only use a desktop. See which works best for you.

- You might get enough distance from the electronics of a laptop by attaching an external keyboard and mouse and useing a larger type font.

Removing Odors from the Outside Casing of Electronics

- Most outside cases or coverings of electronic equipment have oil or some other coating from the manufacturing process. To remove it, use Everclear™ or grain alcohol from a liquor store. If you are sensitive to these, do it outside. Wipe the telephone, keyboard etc. It dries quickly and doesn't ruin the electronics.

- If you are sensitive to VOC emissions from a television set or other electronic item, encase it in a vented box built out of safe wood, metal or glass. If possible, put an exhaust fan and dryer vent hose on the case to take the fumes to an air cleaner or out of the living space.

- Best is to vent the fumes outside of the house. However, except for the very sensitive, if led away from the user, they will oxidize and become nontoxic.

- A small fan blowing the fumes away, work for many.

- If necessary, increase the font size to make reading easier.

- PWCS find used or store display models that have had time to offgass more tolerable, unless they have been saturated with fragrance.

- People seem to have more success with plasma monitors.

- Others have had success with a piece of glass two or three inches in front of the monitor.

- Run new items somewhere away from you for as long as it takes the item to offgass.

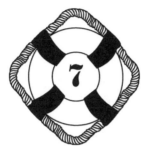

The Kitchen, Bathroom, Garage, and Utility Room

The kitchen, bathroom, garage, and utility room are four areas containing numerous toxins. The culprits reside under sinks, in cabinets, on shelves, the material that the shelves and cabinets are made of, and in corners of the utility rooms, and garage.

Products that are dangerous to your health include common commercial items that most non-CS, and many PWCS in an earlier period of their life, used without problems. A short list includes: cleaners, old paint cans, brushes, solvents, soaps, lotions, art supplies, motorcycles, grease laden bicycles, skate boards, boxes of saved perfumed or moldy letters, photos, pictures that you intend to hang some day, etc. They need to be gathered, sorted, the toxin emitting ones that one thinks will be of some use one day, contained in a closed container. Best would be, if they can be emotionally parted with—thrown away.

Those that you cannot part with for sentimental reasons, or those you need to keep in the hope that some day you may recover enough to use them, are best placed in a covered metal container. Things that you think might be safe and want to bring into your living space can individually be tested. If you find it is safe, bring it back in. Products that are toxic for you, but necessary for daily living or maintaining your home, can generally be replaced with nontoxic substitutes, or stored in a manner that keeps them away from you.

Storage and Testing

- A clean, galvanized garbage can with a cover, works well to store toxic items.

- Clear hard plastic boxes with a good cover also works if not directly in the living space. One can see what is being stored.

- Test large items that you wish to bring into your living space by leaving them in a closed safe room for a while. Then cautiously walk in, take a sniff and observe what happens to you.

- Entering the room slowly, tip of the nose first and limiting your exposure is strongly advised.

- Smaller items can be placed in a closed mason jar for a while and then open it and--smell.[1]

Kitchen

- Turn off all gas/propane appliances at the source.

- There is a simple toggle on the gas line located just behind the stove that, when turned perpendicular to the line, will shut off the gas.

- If you don't want to, the gas company will do it for you.

- It is best that the home of someone who has CS not have ANY gas/propane appliances.

- Best solution--have the gas line completely removed from the house to guard against an accidental leak.

- Electric stoves and ranges are best.

- Sterno™ should never be used.

---

1. When testing an item on yourself, do it very slowly. If you do not have a reaction, you can breathe deeper and longer. Unfortunately, you are the only judge of whether an item is safe or not.

- If food smells are a problem, separate the kitchen from the rest of the house to keep the cooking odors from spreading throughout the home.

- Keep the kitchen under negative pressure with a small exhaust fan or oven hood to help keep food odors, as well as odors from electrical machinery such as refrigerators, from permeating the rest of the house.

- Make sure to install a baffle, or design it in some way that air does not blow back into the house.

- One can purchase and easily install vent sealers that operate electrically. When the fan is turned on, the baffle will open, and close when the fan is turned off.[2]

- Air rises in a house. Odors from a first floor kitchen will find their way into a second story bedroom.

- If necessary, you can build a quick, nontoxic wall to separate an open kitchen from the rest of the house with metal studs, covered with mirror.

- The edges of the mirror can be sealed with silicone if tolerated, or metal tape.

- Do not use the normal black mirror adhesive. It is very toxic. Instead simply have holes drilled in the mirror and screw it into the studs.

- Aluminum channels, to hold the mirrors, are another option.

- Install an exhaust fan or oven hood over the stove that carries the cooking odors outside.

- Seal all wood cabinets with a safe sealer. They are commonly made with chipboard or some other toxic substance.

- If you cannot tolerate any sealer, cover them with aluminum foil and metal tape.

- Best solution-- replace them with safe hardwood or metal.

- Or cover as much as you can with sheet metal.

- Replace chipboard shelves with glass, metal, Formica™, or sealed hardwood.

---

2. Any HVAC company will know how to do this, or the device; under $100 can be purchased from a HVAC supply company.

- Formica™ cabinets and counters are nontoxic if the Formica™ completely covers all six sides and edges and has offgassed.

- If the insides of the cabinets have holes to adjust the shelves, metal tape over the ones not in use as more likely than not the cabinet is chipboard covered with a wood veneer or Formica™, and toxins will leak out of the holes.

- Inspect the underneath of the counter tops. If they are made of chipboard, either seal, or better yet, cover it with aluminum foil and metal tape.

- If any other areas are questionable, your best friends will be aluminum foil and metal tape.

Cooking and Cleanup

- Electric stoves are best. As noted, ALL gas/propane appliances, as noted above, should be turned off at the source.

- Better solution--remove the gas line from the house.

- If gas is needed to supply a downwind, outside grill, run the line along the outside of the house.

- Even outside, cooking with gas/propane is not recommended; the fumes get into the food.

- Charcoal or propane grills should never be used by PWCS, nor food cooked from them eaten.

- If you must cook on gas/propane, do it outside, and place a pan between the food and the flame so that gas fumes do not get into the food.

- Make sure that you are standing up wind of the grill when cooking.

- Electric outdoor grills are available at most appliance stores.

- Glass pots and pans are safest for cooking use.[3]

---

3. Corning™ used to make Vision Wear™, which was made out of heat resistant glass. They no longer make it, but you can usually find some on Ebay.com. Others have reported that they have started to make it again. Amber is the best color to use, as some of the others leech toxins

- Most PWCS prefer Stainless steel cooking utensils.

- Corning makes a fine line of glass pots and pans. Sometimes they are hard to find, but can often be obtained from eBay.com.

- Avoid aluminum, Teflon™, and any coated surface.

- Use non-porous plates and cups and metal silverware.

- Avoid plastics.

- If cooking smells bother you, and you cannot isolate the kitchen, cook on an electric outside grill or on a hot plate in an area separate from the living space, such as a porch, or patio.

- Open a window in the kitchen while exhausting so as not to de-pressurize the house and draw toxins out of the walls.

- Keep an open box of baking soda in the refrigerator and under the sink to absorb odors.

- If you are pesticide sensitive, do not use commercial liquid dishwashing detergent or laundry detergent as they all contain fungicides.

- Many who are not pesticide sensitive tolerate Seventh Generation™ dish liquid and powdered dishwashing detergent.

- Powdered detergent is best, as many liquid detergents contain fungacides..

- Baking soda is an alternative to a detergent in the dishwasher.

- Bon Ami™ is a good abrasive cleanser. It does not contain chlorine, perfume or dye.

- Stainless steel or copper scrubbing pads without additives can be purchased at most super markets.

- Do not use commercial oven cleaners.

- If you live in an apartment building and your kitchen does not have a window, it might be connected to an airshaft that allows the odors from other peoples apartments to come into yours.

---

into the food.

- If this is true, either cover it up, or install an exhaust fan in the opening to the airshaft.

- You can tell if air is coming in through the vent or going out by simply holding up a thin strip of tissue and watching what happens to it.

Bathroom

- Keep the bathroom as clean and dry as possible to prevent mold growth.

- Keep dirty laundry in a covered container, or separate room.

- Good airflow will keep the bathroom dry.

- Mold grows best in dark, warm, wet, places with something to feed on.

- Other than towels, the bathroom should not contain any soft goods such as curtains, window shades, wall paper, pillows, etc.

- Cotton throw rugs are fine if washed often.

- Metal aluminum blinds are nontoxic.

- Install and run at low speed 24/7, a bathroom exhaust fan.

- If you can tolerate a nylon shower curtain, it is better than cotton as it dries faster and will not grow mold if kept clean.

- If the shower is large enough, you can get away without a shower curtain by using towels on the floor in front of the shower.

- If you use a shower curtain, leave it open after it dries to air out the shower and prevent mold build up.

- Wash the shower curtain often.

- If you are building a new home or remodeling the bathroom, grade a tiled floor downwards toward the shower drain and you will never need a curtain. To wash, you just squeegee the water toward the drain.

- Keep all bathroom cleaning and cosmetic items behind closed doors or in a separate closed room.

- If you live in an apartment building, and the bathroom does not have a window, your bathroom is most likely vented to a common exhaust well connected to all the other bathrooms, in the building. This means that "smelly stuff" from other peoples bathrooms are flowing into your space. Cover the vent or install an exhaust fan in it.

- As noted above, you can check the air trough this vent by holding a thin piece of tissue over it and observing which way it is fluttering.

- Bathroom grout can be kept mold free by washing it with a brush dipped in hydrogen peroxide, vinegar, or Bon Ami™.

- A steamer, as noted below, is nontoxic, inexpensive, and works well to clean and prevent mold buildup.

- If you use a steamer, it is safest to make your own pads from old towels. You can discard them after use to avoid mold growth.

- Keep an open box of baking soda in the bathroom to absorb odors.

The Garage and Utility Room

- If the garage is attached to the house, empty it of any chemical products.

- Find and remove old paint cans, used brushes, gasoline cans, gasoline powered mowers, trimmers, leaf blowers, motor oil, cleaning supplies, etc.

- Discard any that the PWCS needs to avoid, when possible.

- Use metal cabinets, or hard covered plastic boxes to store any items that need to be kept, or those in use.

- Store things you need to keep in a storage shed, downwind from the house.

- Better--sell them on Ebay and use the money to hire a lawn service.

- Wash old oil spills off of the garage floor with Tri Sodium Phosphate (TSP), which needs hot water to activate.[4]

---

4. TSP is available at most hardware stores. Follow the directions. Even though it is not corrosive or toxic to most, wear gloves, goggles, and rinse well.

- Do not park your car, or lawn mower, or any gasoline powered machinery in an attached garage, especially one that is on the lower level, as the fumes will find their way into the house.

- If the garage is located on the side of the house, the wall between the garage and house can, and should be sealed.

- Better--the car will be just fine outside. Think of it as driveway jewelry.

- If snow is a problem, a snow shed or car port can easily be constructed.

- Devices are available to keep the engine warm in very cold climates, or a separate heated garage might have to be constructed.

- Keep the garage and utility room, if attached to the house, under negative pressure to prevent toxins from items that will ultimately be stored there, or air leaks from leaching into the living space.

- To do this, simply install an exhaust fan in a window or through the wall.

- Install an airtight door between the garage and house.

- Best—thoroughly seal the garage from the rest of the house. Pay careful attention to the seams, pipes and wires that go through the ceiling or walls.

Furnace

- If the furnace must be kept in the house, wall it off in a well-sealed room, vented to the outside.

- Talk to an HVAC person about the proper way to exhaust a room that contains the furnace, as it might interfere with its operation.

Exercise Room or Area

- Everyone knows that exercise is important for health, and for PWCS it also helps metabolize stored toxins, so if devise a plan if possible.

- Walking in a safe area is the cheapest way to exercise.

- New exercise equipment, not recommended, contains rubber and plastic.

- Generally they will offgass over time.

- The rubber parts can be covered with aluminum foil and metal tape.

- The motors might give off ozone or some other toxic substance.

- Used exercise equipment might be offgassed enough for most.

- Test used equipment before you buy.

- Old Nordic Track™ cross-country ski machines, are mechanical, do not contain rubber or plastic and are made out of hardwood. They are available from time to time on eBay.com and can be cleaned up.

- For the very sensitive, free metal weights are nontoxic, and cheaper.

- Used, non-computerized, mechanical exercise bikes are nontoxic.

- Swimming is great exercise.

- Do not swim in a pool using chlorine or chemicals to clean the water.

- Non-chlorinated pools are hard to find but available in many areas.

- If you live near the ocean or a lake, you have a perfect situation.

- If you already own a pool, discuss salt free methods of sanitization with a pool expert. There are many options available.

- Send a sample of water from a lake you'd like to swim in to a testing lab.

- Buy and offgass a wet suit for a year or so. If lucky, you might be able to swim all year in colder climates. If not, resell it on eBay.

- Offgass the wet suit it by leaving it outdoors or at least in sunny airy place.

- Some wetsuits are lined with a material or wool which may be tolerated.

- For some, wearing long cotton underwear, under the suit might be protection enough from the wet suit.

- Caution! Although the above sounds good, not everyone can tolerate even well offgassed Neoprene™ as it is made from petrochemicals.

General Cleaners

- Most commercial cleaning products, even the ones marked "fragrance free", "green", or "natural", contain perfume or other chemical ingredients.

- A steamer works wonderfully for non-porous floors. It kills mold, is nontoxic and does not use any chemicals.

- A steamer will also kill any mold build-up in humid, bathrooms and showers.

- Floor steamers, and hand steamers are available.

- Some hand steamers have plastic hoses and may not be as well tolerated as the floor steamer. They tend to be difficult to offgass.

- Some steamers have attachments that allow you to clean walls, mirrors, furniture, windows, and even the hubcaps of your car.

- Baking soda is a wonderful cleaner and deodorizer with innumerable uses.

- Use vinegar if tolerated.

- Use common rubbing alcohol if tolerated.

- Use Super Clean™ if tolerated.[5]

- Use Shaklee's Basic™ if tolerated.

- Bon Ami™ is a good nontoxic scouring powder.

- Hydrogen peroxide will clean, bleach grout, and kill mold. Only use food grade peroxide if well diluted.[6]

- Micro-fiber™ cloths from "Solutions" catalogue.[7]

- Use plain, soap free steel scrubbing pads.

- Grapefruit seed extract will sterilize counters.

---

5. http://freshrv.com/supercleans.aspx. It cleans rugs, upholstery, sweaters, clothes, windows, and many other things.

6. Use gloves if using food grade hydrogen peroxide.

7. 1-888-55MICRO, microfibertech.com

- Vinegar and baking soda will clear up clogged drains. Put baking soda down drains; pour in vinegar and close stopper. Let it bubble and fizz a while, then run water through.

Glass and Window Cleaner

- A spray bottle filled with a mixture of Super Clean™[8] and water. You can add vinegar if tolerated.

- Earth Friendly Window Kleener™[9]

- 70% alcohol works well, and kills everything, if you can tolerate it.

- Some hand steamers have window/mirror washing attachments.

Dish Washing

- Hot water.

- Granny's EZ Maid™.[10]

- Seventh Generation Free and Clear™.[11]

Household Paper Goods

- Use well washed cotton cloths and towels.

- Use paper products that do not have any scents, printing, patterns, or additives.

- Do not purchase paper products that are stored near the cleaning or other smelly products in the store as they will absorb the odors.

- If you find they are smelly, air them out, or try another brand.

---

8. Most places that sell products for the sensitive, such as the Environmental Health Center in Dallas, 214- 368-4132, www.ehcd.com.

9. IBID

10. Available at most places that sell products for the environmentally sensitive.

11. IBID.

Garbage Containers

- Use a covered porcelain pail.

- Use galvanized metal garbage cans.

- Some plastic garbage bags smell as the manufacturer adds something, to disquise the smell of garbage. Some products change every so often.

- As of this writing, Hefty™ garbage bags do not contain additional odors. Also, Wegman's own brand seems to have no odor at this time.

- Hydrogen peroxide will clean, bleach grout, and kill mold.[12]

Removing Odors from Your Hands

- Rub your hands with a stainless steel soupspoon, or a piece of stainless steel, while holding them under warm water.

- Amco makes a stainless steel soap shaped bar called "Rub-A-Way".

- Lemon.

- Baking Soda.

---

12. Use gloves if using food grade hydrogen peroxide.

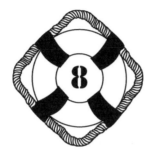

Personal Care Products

Personal care products, which include items such as cosmetics, clothing, soaps, shampoos, conditioners, hair coloring, deodorants, and laundry products, can be an important source of toxins. They enter the body through the nose, mouth, of the skin, the body's largest organ.

It has been estimated that five pounds of cosmetic ingredients enter a woman's body each year. Many of the ingredients of these products are not listed on the label. They are not tested for safety, and the effects of combining these chemicals on the human body are unknown. This might possibly explain why more woman report CS symptoms than men as they tend to use more personal products than men.[1]

Great care should be taken by anyone using these products to use them as little as possible, and to select the safest product you can find. This can be difficult because the words "natural", hypoallergenic,

---

1. This is not a sexist statement. For whatever reason, women have been studied more than men in this illness. Jonathon Morgan, "Woman's Bodies May Absorb Five Pounds of Makeup Chemicals Per Year." Telegraphco.uk, July 19, 2007. As noted in a previous chapter, it is not proven that more women get MCS than men, as more women have been surveyed than men.

or organic do not equate to their being safe for a PWCS. They are more likely a marketing device created by the personal care industry as more and more of the population becomes conscious of the health hazards of the so called "safe" stuff they are rubbing on their skin, eating off their lips, and breathing into their lungs all day.

Most of the commercial so-called "safe" products do contain perfumes, coloring and chemicals; even those sold in so called health food stores. Many products are labled as "Natural" because they contain natural ingredients, however that does not mean that they are safe for everyone. Read the labels, questionable products should either be tested or avoided. The following contains products and suggestions from the readership of *Our Toxic Times*. If you choose to try using one of them, as with any product, test it first on yourself, as what everyone tolerates is different.[1]

Soaps:[2]

- Glycerin soap.

- Eucerin Pump Soap.

- DHC Mild Soap. [3]

- Magick Botanicals has a number of products.[4]

- Chef's Soap.

- Simple Soap.

- Kiss My Face Soap.

- Rokeach's Kosher Kitchen bar soap.

---

2. If you find one that is safe for you, it is wise to stockpile a supply as formulas often change without notice. Most of the products mentioned can be obtained from Janice's 1-800-Janice, Needs, or the Environmental Health Center in Dallas. Johnson and Johnson also makes a sensitive skin fragrance free group of products. They are hard to find but can be obtained from the company.

3. 1-800-DHC care.

4. Magick Botanicals, 1-800-237-0674 has a number of products.

Tooth Paste:

- Baking Soda and sea salt mixture. Dip a wet toothbrush in the mixture.

- Baking Soda and hydrogen peroxide paste.

- Tom's of Maine makes toothpaste without fluoride and a natural baking soda product without additives.

- 1-888-Eco-dent makes effervescent baking soda toothpaste but it has other ingredients, therefore, it must be tested.

Shampoo:

- Stony ~~Brode~~ *Brook* Botanier[5]

- Goats milk shampoo and soap from Dionis[6]

has parabens; are going to discontinue product

Deodorant:

- Soap and water. is best. Odors from a clean body are natural. It is the bacteria that smells, not you. Perfume companies attempt to duplicate natural body odors to increase our attractiveness.[7]

- Crystal deodorant stones, if you must wear deodorant at all.[8]

- A small amount of baking soda applied to a damp area of skin.

---

5. Stony Brode Botanier, Rainbow Research, 170 Wilbur Place, Bohemia, NY 11716.

6. Dionis, 1-800-566-7627.

7. A pungent smell coming out of your body does not mean that you are "smelly" and thus unlovable. The odor is probably due to the chemicals that your body is removing. When you put a deodorant on, you stop the sweating process and prevent your body from detoxifying. Although highly speculative, I wonder if this covering up of our natural odors designed to attract compatible people is part of the reason for the high divorce rate in the United States.

8. Many places sell these. Try NEEDS, 1-800-634-1380, www.needs.com.

Cosmetics:

The natural look is best for PWCS, but if you feel you must use cosmetics, here are some suggestions, at the risk of redundancy, test first:[9]

- Ecco Bella

- Clinique.

- Kiehls.[10]

- Lancome, foundation and mascara. (Some PWCS can use.)

- Aveda.

- Bare Essentials.[11]

- Black mascara has fewer ingredients than colored mascara.

- Hain Pure Foods[12] Apricot Kernel Oil or Almond Oil make wonderful moisturizers.

Sunscreen:

- If you must use one, "unscented" or "natural" is not good enough. Most sunscreens contain chemicals. However, some are better than others. You may have to try many to try and find one that will work for you. Unscented may be sufficient for you to be around others who will be wearing it.

- Better is to wear a large "safe" hat and stay covered up.

- Purchase white "sunscreen" clothing from Lands End.

---

9. Many chemically sensitive people cannot tolerate any cosmetics. The less chemically sensitive can tolerate some. These suggestions are offered as possible choices and more so, for non-CS significant others.

10. Kiehls, 1-800-kiehls-1. They will send you free samples.

11..Bare Essentials, 1-800-345-4492.

10. Kiehls, 1-800-kiehls-1. They will send you free samples.

Hair Coloring:

- Commercial products are never good for a PWCS.

- If you are not that sensitive you might get away with Aveda™, which has worked for some.

- If your non-CS significant other must use hair coloring, try Aveda™, have them sleep in another room for a few days, and wear a barrier cloth cap if in bed with you.[13] Test First!

- Some people report success with Henna or the natural tints from Health food stores.

Hairspray:

- Two cups of boiling water, 1 tsp. Knox gelatin, 1 tsp. lemon. Mix and filter. Stay away from bugs at picnics.

Removing Outside Odors from Your Hair:

- Wash well.

- Use a hair dryer, one that has an ionizing setting if tolerable.

- Wash your hair in baking soda.

- Air out, drive home with the window down, and stay outside a while.

---

12. Aveda, 1-866-823-1423, www.aveda.com. If having Aveda applied professionally, afterwards, have the salon wash three times, with unscented shampoo. Have person sleep in separate bedroom for two days, or until their hair stops smelling. A barrier cloth hair bonnet helps when they come back into the same bed with you and the residual odor on their hair still bothers you.

Clothing:

Clothing can bother PWCS. It touches the skin, which can absorb any toxins in the material. If it is a synthetic fabric, it is made from petrochemicals. Even 100 per cent cotton fabric is often coated with another chemical to make it wrinkle-free and stain resistant. It may also contain chemicals used in the bleaching or coloring process. If it is "dry clean only", it emits toxins from the chemicals used to clean it.

- 100% well washed cotton in neutral tones.[14]

- Newly purchased cotton clothing needs to be washed a few times in baking soda, and/or TSP before wearing to remove any chemicals and odors picked up in the manufacturing process, or from being in a formaldehyde laden store.[15]

- Some people have found that soaking the article of clothing in milk works to remove odors.

- Recycled or used sometimes works, but, smell before you buy.

- If you still have trouble with well-washed cotton, air it out and expose it to the sun as long as necessary, but clothes left in the sun too long will begin to fade, so check them often.

- This might also work with synthetic fibers if you are not too sensitive.

- Silk, if you can tolerate the odor.

- Linen, if it does not have any additives.

- Wool or blends, if tolerated. Do not dry-clean, after wearing air out and brush.

- Some wool without lining can be washed, but it has a strong odor when wet and as it ages. Wetting can also reactivate old smells and make it no longer tolerable for you.

- Synthetic or wool outerwear, if it is old and well offgassed.

---

13. Cotton is a miracle fiber. It is cool in the summer, warm in the winter if layered. In addition, cotton can be washed at home, as dry cleaning anything is very bad. Some prefer organic, others do not. This is an individual choice, and you will need to test both.

14. TSP is readily available at most hardware stores. TSP needs to be mixed in hot water to activate.

- Layered cotton outerwear is best.

- If you must dry clean an item of clothing, find a nontoxic dry cleaner and even then, after you pick them up, air them out very well in a separate space for a long time before you use them again.[16]

- Many people keep a clothesline outside, and/or a separate space in the home for this purpose.

- Stretch fabrics, (contain rubber) and synthetics are usually not well tolerated, and unless well tested should be avoided.

- Treated clothes, permanent press, wrinkle free etc., are a problem for many PWCS as they are treated with polyester, formaldehyde, pesticides, or Teflon to make them easy care or mold resistant. Many of these toxic ingredients are impossible to remove.

- A pressure cooker will pull soaps and chemicals out of used clothes. Pour off liquid outside, not in your sink. Do not use the cooker for food after this.

- If all of the above suggestions do not work, donate them or throw them away.

- Better yet, sell them on eBay.

Shoes:

- Safe shoes are difficult to find, and are a very individualistic choice.

- Best shoes are those that can be washed.

- Cotton shoes are available from yoga supply stores, but usually need lots of washing.

- All new shoes smell.

- Older shoes are best.

- Leather insoles are better than synthetic.

---

15. Perchlorethylene, the dry cleaning solvent is very toxic, proven by the high cancer rate of individuals that work in the industry.

- Try them on for size at home if the store has a return policy.

- Buy shoes in advance so they can outgas before you need to wear them.

- If the shoes have inserts, remove and outgas shoe and insert separately. Preferably outside, or in a space separate from your living space, and/or near a source of sunlight light and heat.

- Old-fashioned canvas sneakers work for some people.

- Use Huggies Supreme Care™ fragrance free baby wipes to polish shoes.

Laundry:

- Wash and dry your clothes at home, preferably in a new machine that has porcelain or stainless drums and inside case. Obviously, plastic or composite materials should be avoided.

- If the machine is old and has been used with "smelly" stuff, run it a few times with baking soda and TSP to remove the odors.

- It is better to dry clothes in an electric dryer, than in polluted outside air where they will pick up free floating odors, air pollution particles, and pollen.

- Baking soda and borax work for general washing needs.

- Arm and Hammer™ fragrance free detergent works for some.

- Detergents sold in stores that cater to PWCS people can be tried, but be cautious, many claim to be natural, but contain fragrance and other ingredients to make them more marketable.

- Use powdered detergents, as liquid ones, even the so called green ones, contain fungicides.

- If very sensitive, just use water.

- For stains try: Hydrogen peroxide, (applied directly to the stain) or one cup per load.

- Try Oxyclean™, or lemon juice. You may have to mix with detergent.

- Always test a patch of the fabric in a hidden area first.

- Some people tolerate a bleach stick, applied by someone else.

- If you are able to wear polyester clothes or other synthetic materials, you can add a cup of vinegar to the wash and it will help with wrinkles and static electricity, instead of using fabric softeners.

- To remove wrinkles, put the clothes in the dryer just long enough to heat them up, and then hang them to dry—no, or very little ironing is needed and this method doesn't wear clothes out as quickly.

- Never leave wet clothes in the washing machine; mold or mildew may grow.

- Always leave the washing machine door open when not in use to keep it dry and prevent mold growth.

- Throw some baking soda into the washing machine when not in use to prevent possible mold growth in any water that might remain. When you run the washer, the baking soda will dissolve.

Removing Odors in New Cloths and Bedding:

- Soak clothes in full fat milk as you want the butterfat in the milk to absorb the fat soluble chemicals, for a couple of hours to release the toxins.

- Wash many times in warm water containing TSP, baking soda and borax.

- Vinegar.

- Oxyclean™.

Removing Odors from Clothes
That Have Been Worn Outside or in Public Places:

- Put in dryer for 40 minutes at high, (not wool as it must be dried naturally).

- Use a hair dryer, the ones that ionize work best.

- Air out on a clothesline in the sun for as long as necessary.

- Leave for a few days in a place that is separated from your living space.

- If the article of clothing doesn't air out in a reasonable time, it is a candidate for eBay.

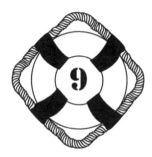

Finding a Safe Automobile

Finding a safe, non-symptom producing automobile is one of the more challenging problems facing people with Multiple Chemical Sensitivity–a necessity in modern America.

The reasons that it is very difficult to obtain a "safe" automobile are inherent in the nature of the machine. An automobile is constructed of numerous, potentially toxic ingredients such as glues, sealers, plastics, rubber, and Scotch Guard™ type applications on fabric seats, synthetic fibers, tanned leather, hidden sound proofing material, and other items known, unknown, and unknowable. In addition, the vehicle itself contains substantial quantities of oil, antifreeze, refrigerant, lubricant, and gasoline that may leak, but surely emit toxic fumes as the vehicle runs and can enter the passenger compartment.[1]

---

1. Gas powered vehicles are infinitely safer than those that use diesel fuel. Scotch Guard™ is under investigation for emitting toxic fumes and is being discontinued after years of use. The EPA recently released the following statement: "PFOS The ingredient in Scotch Guard™ is of significant concern on the basis of evidence of widespread human exposure and indications of toxicity. These chemicals "combine persistence, bioaccumulation, and toxicity properties to an extraordinary degree." (EPA internal memorandum, May 16, 2000.)

The automobile also travels on roads where its air intake can "inhale" toxic fumes through openings in its body or fresh air ventilation system; fumes emitted from other vehicles, tarred roads, or free floating air pollution. Some manufacturers, General Motors in particular, in spite of increasing evidence that materials in automobiles are toxic to all people, add substances to the vehicle to maintain that "new car" smell that non-CS buyers seem to like. Some used car dealers add it, or other odiferous chemicals, to their used cars to increase their appeal and cover up bad smells from previous occupants.

To further complicate an already difficult issue, there is no guarantee that a particular "brand" either: recommended by others; used successfully by you in the past; or advertised as environmentally safe; will this time, be safe for you. Materials used in the automobile can change without notice. The same vehicle and model might be manufactured in different countries where local materials are used increasing the chances that each vehicle might be different. And as always with this illness, what is safe for one can be toxic for another.[2]

The project is critical, daunting, but not hopeless. Surprisingly, most PWCS have successfully solved it and found a safe enough car to drive. This chapter will give general guidelines to give you the best chances of obtaining such a vehicle. How far one has to go in order to achieve this depends on one's sensitivities, and the vehicle.[3] As with everything else in this illness, a "safe" car is a very personal matter and the final choice must be individually tested and approved by you.

- A good place to start is http://press.healthystuff.org/departments/cars/index.php.

- Cautiously smell any vehicle you are considering before you purchase.

- Top of the line, most expensive automobiles tends to be made with more care and of better materials and thus have a better chance of success.[4]

---

2. Some manufacturers, Volvo and BMW come to mind, advertise that they only use "green" environmentally safe material in their products. What is green for them has not been green for me. It took three years before I could ride in my wife's Volvo, and even after five years when my brother-in-law was trading in his BMW, I was unable to tolerate it. Recently I heard that Toyota was developing a vehicle manufactured from "safe" ingredients, but as of yet there have not been any reports favorable or unfavorable. A reader reports using a new Honda™ after only 3 months.

3. Contact the Human Ecology Action League, 404-248-1898, healnatnl@aol.com for reprints of articles that they have published on the subject of making a car safe.

4. For example, quality shoes are stitched, cheaper ones glued.

- If you purchase a new car from a new car dealer, look for the one out that has been on lot the longest time.[5]

- The older the vehicle, the greater chance, not guarantee, of success for the materials to have offgassed. However, the length of time needed can vary greatly.

- Used cars may not follow this rule as previous owners may have made the car toxic beyond fixing.

- Check with your friends and relatives that do not routinely use fragrance or smoke. Perhaps you can purchase their car.

- Smell all of your friends and relative's cars to give you a sense of which manufacturers and year to consider, or avoid. Remember each year and model may be different.

- Some people have found a good, nontoxic car on a used car dealer's lot.

- Simply go from vehicle to vehicle, smell, or sit in them and see what happens to you.[6]

- Turn on the heating and air conditioning system, and smell the air coming out of the vents. HVAC systems tend to hold odors and are difficult to clean.

- Stay away from any used car that has that smelly little green tree, or any other air freshener, hanging from the mirror. Don't even go in it.

- Purchase a "certified" used car from a reputable dealer in order to obtain a long warrantee. Many manufacturers extend the warrantee up to 100,000 miles on their "certified" used cars.

- A certified pre-owned vehicle can be bought for less money than a new one, comes with a longer bumper to bumper guarantee, and has had time for the leather, vinyl, rubber gaskets, etc. to have offgassed.

- If you chose this method, ask the dealer whether or not they routinely or have recently detailed the vehicle.

---

5. The date of manufacture can easily be obtained from the dealer or the VIN number.

6. One reader reported that she was able to find a safe used Ford by walking through a dealer's lot and sitting in car after car time and time again until she found one.

- Tell the dealer what you are looking for and to call you when one comes in before they clean it, so you can test it.

- If you are ordering in a new car, ask the dealer not to detail the inside before you pick it up.

- Purchase a new car well in advance of when you intend to use it to allow offgassing time.

- Better, let a friend or relative who does not use perfume or smelly deodorant drive it until it offgasses.

- If you purchase a new vehicle, pay extra for an extended warrantee, as once it becomes safe, you will want to keep it as long as possible.

- Only purchase an extended warrantee from the manufacturer of the vehicle. Third party ones tend to be scams.

- Cloth seats offgass better than vinyl or leather.

- Expensive leather offgasses better than cheap leather.

- Some leather may never offgass. It depends on the quality and what chemicals were used to tan it.

- If possible, buy a car that has "lived" for a while, preferably un-detailed on dealer's lot, in a hot, dry, desert state such as Arizona. The reasons are obvious.

- Think convertible. Unlike years ago, the better ones are very air tight, and you can leave the top down in the sun, or open in a garage, to speed up the offgassing time.

- UV light and air are excellent aids in speeding up the offgassing time.

- Even if the top does not go down, leave the car in the sun as much as possible to heat up the material on the inside.

- Sunroofs are helpful in this process. A car with a sunroof is a good way to let UV light into the vehicle when not in use.

- If you are letting the sun heat the car and speed up offgassing time, make sure to leave a window open a crack so the toxic fumes can escape, rather than be reabsorbed.

- Another option is to leave the car in a well-ventilated garage with the car doors open for as long as necessary.

- If you do this, disconnect the automatic door open light, either by a switch, or remove the fuse.

- Leaving the doors open will also help offgass the door gaskets. Disengage the interior lights that go on when the door is open so you can leave the door open when the weather warrants it and you are not using it. This will offgass the rubber gaskets on the doors.

- Try a combination of heat, humidity, and leaving an open box of baking soda in the vehicle to shorten offgassing time.

- Try an ionizing hair dryer on the leather, cloth, and vinyl surfaces of the vehicle.

- Washing all vinyl surfaces with: apple cider vinegar, and/or Supercleans™ have worked for some.[7]

- Washing smelly areas with a solution of baking soda in water, and/or TSP has also worked for some.

- Success has been reported by washing fabric seats with Mystical™.[8]

- Success has been reported with a product called Odor Eliminator™.[9]

- Cover seats that still smell with cotton seat covers.

- If necessary, wrap them first in medical grade Tyvek™ and barrier cloth.

- Cover all other exposed problem areas with medical grade Tyvek™, and barrier cloth.

- If necessary obtain a diagram from the manufacturer in order to remove things like dashboards, sun visors, and door panels. Wash, thoroughly air out, cover and replace.

- The less smelly material in the car to make you sick, the better.

- Discard all floor mats, as they are rubber based.

---

7. http://www.supercleans.com/

8. This can be purchased from any store that caters to PWCS, such as Janice's, N.EE.D.S. etc.

9. Odor Eliminator can be purchased from Target.

- If necessary, remove the floor carpeting under the mats. Live with bare metal while the carpeting is offgassing in a separate space or permanently if necessary.

- Save them, you can put them back when you are ready to sell the car and they will make it look newer.

- Go one step further and remove everything that can be removed, the end point being bare metal.

- Bare metal should be washed with TSP to remove oil or other toxins remaining from the manufacturing process.

- The removed items can be left in the sun or a warm place with good airflow until they become nontoxic and then reinstalled.

- Most of them just snap in, but a manufacturer's diagram is needed unless you are very handy or familiar with automobiles.

- Make sure the vehicle you purchase has an air filtration system that can be closed off to outside air.

- If the vehicle cannot permanently shut off outside air, have a mechanic alter it by changing the settings, or if necessary closing off the air intake.

- Some vehicles say that the vents can be closed to the recirculation position, but open periodically open and let fresh air in as the manufacturer is trying to guard against a carbon monoxide leak. You should know this and decide whether or not to let a mechanic change it.

- If you do this, periodically open and close a window to prevent any carbon monoxide build up.

- Some vehicles come with HEPA and charcoal air filtration systems.

- Purchase a spare filter and leave it exposed to the air so the manufacturing odor will have offgassed by the time you need to replace it.

- Try a charcoal/HEPA automobile air filter, available from NEEDS or E.L. Faust.

- Do not use any filtration system that produces ions or ozone.

- Keep a portable oxygen tank in the car for emergencies, or to drive a car that has not yet offgassed.

- Do not fill the gas tank yourself. Ask the attendant to do it and give him a tip. Check for wind direction first and pull up to a pump so that the wind will blow the fumes away from your vehicle.

- If possible, purchase a vehicle that has the gas cap on the passenger side.

- When you replace the tires, let some one else drive the car for a day or so to burn off the new rubber smell.

- If you take the car to a car wash, do not let them clean the inside or wax the outside. Vacuum it, as long as the attendant is not wearing fragrance.

- Do not wax or detail the outside of the vehicle, the fumes, especially when heated by the sun, are toxic, will get into the car.

- Choose car washes that you drive the vehicle through or where it is pulled through by a machine, rather than let some unknown individual with smelly stuff on drive it and make it toxic.

- Always park it yourself, even if the sign says "valet" parking. Simply hand the attendant a dollar and tell them that you will park it. A dollar goes a long way.

- When you service the vehicle, cover the seats with plastic bags, cover the steering wheel with aluminum foil, and tell the dealer not to clean the inside, as some dealers automatically include a car wash and cleaning as part of the service.

- If you have found a "safe" car, keep it as long as you possibly can, or at least until a replacement is ready.

- Check consumer guide for vehicles with the lowest repair history to increase your chances of keeping the car for a long time.

- If you keep the car for a long time, change the hoses after 100,000 miles whether they need it or not. Otherwise the vehicle is an accident waiting to happen.

- Obviously, keep it in good repair.

- If you are repurchasing the same brand of vehicle that you are trading in, see if the seats from the old vehicle will fit in the new one.

Sometimes they do and switching them out will save you lots of offgassing time and grief.

- The dealer will be happy to put your new seats in the used car.

- If the dealer balks, a few dollars given to the service manager might do the trick.

- Electric windows are handy to close the car up quickly or release toxins.

- When you leave the car, leave the ventilation system open (on fresh air) to keep it dry, mold free, and give the vehicle some air circulation when not in use.

- Some people have reported success by ozonating a car for twenty-four hours and then letting it air out for a few days.

- Be careful, ozone is very toxic to people and rubber components of the vehicle. The above strategy should be professionally done.

- Have a mechanic check a used car not only for its mechanics, but also or any exhaust leaks.

- Have a mechanic also look over the vehicle for any possible leaks in the structure that might allow engine, or road fumes to enter the vehicle. These can easily be sealed.

- Some automobiles emit a strong EMF and can get people who are sensitive to EMF, sick. This cannot be fixed other than by getting rid of the vehicle.

- Do not park the car in an attached garage.

- If ypu must park the car in an attached garage, wait a few minutes before closing the garage door to allow any exhaust fumes to dissipate.

- If the car is parked in a detached garage to offgass, do not store any odor emitting machinery, such as lawn mowers, gas cans, or chemicals, in the same space.

- By trial, error, perseverance, and luck, most PWCS have obtained a "safe" vehicle.

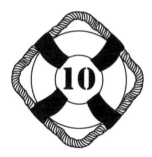

Managing Temporary Time Limited Exposures

This chapter will relate methods that respondents to the OTT survey use to manage temporary, time limited exposures. Obviously, the ability to do this can increase one's time in the world, around people and things that might cause physical symptoms. How much each person can handle is obviously dependent on the usual factors: individual health, type of exposure, and length of time exposed. Unfortunately unwanted, unsought exposures are often unavoidable and strategies have to be in pace in advance to deal with them in the best way possible. Everyone with this illness is different, and reacts to or is helped by different things. What works for one may not work for another.

These suggestions are not intended to be a substitute for medical advice, nor does this book advocate needlessly exposing one's self to potentially damaging toxins. The suggestions in this chapter are predicated on the supposition that you are living in a clean enough house in a clean enough environment. The strategies that follow are not given as a substitute for this. They are passed along for your consideration, as a general philosophy of how to manage the illness and a point of discussion with your physician.

Managing an Unexpected Exposure

- A calm mental state and positive attitude are very important.

- A calm mental state activates the parasympathetic nervous system that promotes healing, or at the very least does not damage the system as the sympathetic (fight or flight) might.

- Therefore, if caught in bad situation, do not panic. Panic activates the sympathetic nervous system, (the "flight or fight" reaction), causing it to release chemicals internally which will make the symptoms worse.

- Fight the urge to get angry or give someone a life lesson. They will not listen. And if they do listen, most likely they will not hear. The only thing your anger will accomplish will be to delay your recovery.

- Forgive them; they know not what effect they are having on you and possibly themselves.

- Convert your anger to political action that might help.

- You cannot control what happens to you. The only thing any of us can control is how we handle it.

- If you have trouble controlling your anger, train a significant other to calm you down. Sometimes, a simple hand on your shoulder or some other agreed upon signal will do it.

- If you don't have a significant other or good friend to call, you must be your own.

- Talk to yourself, as one would to a child to calm your self down. It is the primitive, self-preserving part of you that is reacting.

- Remind yourself that you have been exposed before and recovered. You are still here. There is no reason to think that you will not recover again.

- Change your mental channel. Divert yourself.

- If you cannot divert yourself, go into the pain that the exposure is causing.

- Take slow shallow breaths as you can calmly move away.

- Always be aware of the wind direction, so you can get up wind of an unexpected toxin.

- Practice as much meditation as possible to train the system to maintain it's calm. Breath meditation is particularly good, as is "mindfulness."[1]

- Watch a funny movie, or listen to a humorous tape, for the same reason.

- If you are in a public place or a restaurant and someone wearing "Eau de Harlot", or the worst underarm deodorant you have ever smelled walks past, remember that as they move further away and sit down, the odor will settle, and most likely be contained to where they are. Therefore, you may not have to run out.

- If it does not settle in a few minutes, change your seat.

- Keep a tolerated charcoal mask or respirator with you, ready to put on until you are able to remove yourself from the source of the toxin. Just knowing it is there might help you extend your activities in the world.

- Hold your breath if possible until the source of toxin has passed or you have been able to remove yourself from it

- Obviously at some point you must breathe. When you do so, breathe as shallowly and slowly as you safely can.

- Get fresh air as soon as calmly possible, e.g., leave a toxic restaurant.

- If you are carrying oxygen, use it.

- When you get home, spend time in your clean room. This will allow your body to detoxify.

- Some people argue that going to bed is not advised unless there is no other choice.

- If you are suddenly having symptoms in your safe house, note that your house, which was safe yesterday, did not suddenly get toxic without a reason.

- Your symptoms are probably due to something you ate, or a delayed reaction from a previous exposure.

- Your symptoms could also be detoxing due to entering your clean house after being exposed to whatever.

---

1. Meditation also promotes the parasympathetic (healing) nervous system response. See: Jon Kabat-Zinn, *Wherever You Go, There You Are: Mindfulness in Every Day Life*, NY: Hyperion, 2005.

- Keep a diary to remind yourself of past exposures, how long it took you to recover and what helped you to do so.

- Exercise in a clean space. This helps the body metabolize any stored chemicals.

- Walking fast or exercising after an exposure will also help the body metabolize chemicals from an exposure before they get into your tissues.

- Go to the ocean or salt water if possible.

- Ocean air is usually clean as there is usually an on-shore breeze near the salt water, which contains positive ions that make people feel better.

- Ocean air also contains innumerable minerals that will be absorbed by your skin and utilized by your body.

- This may not be true in some places at low tide, where residue has washed up and is rotting.

- Go in the water, salt water helps the body eliminate toxins and again absorb minerals.

- Or just lie on the beach.

- Find high ground, as the air is usually cleaner the higher one goes.[2]

- Sometimes you can find "clean" air inside a "Jersey" style diner at off hours. These establishments tend to have excellent air systems and are constructed of mostly glass, marble, tile, and Formica.

- Obviously this solution will not work if they are cleaning the diner.

- Some people find large doses of Vitamin C helpful.

- To help the body detox as best as possible, maintain adequate levels of Vitamin C in your system.

- Vitamin C levels change according to body's needs.

- To ascertain the proper level of Vitamin C use a Perque C Strip™ dipped in your urine daily, preferably in the morning.[3]

---

2. Very high altitudes may not be advisable for individuals with respiratory conditions.

3. Available at Needs, Key Pharmacy and other such places.

- Carbohydrates tend to stop some reactions.

- Put your system into an alkaline state with an Alka Seltzer Gold™ or Tri Salts™.

- Some success has been reported with nasal glutathione and nasal, or sublingual hydroxycobalamine.[4]

- Some people report help with sublingual Perque Activated B-12 Guard™.[5]

- Neutralizing doses of Serotonin and Histamine.[6]

- As soon as possible, shower, wash your hair, and change your clothes.

- Dry your hair with an ionizing hair dryer.

- Take a sauna.

- You might get sick in the middle of the sauna, as the toxins leave your body, but will feel better afterwards. The sauna prevents toxin build up.

- If tolerated, old-fashioned aspirin, preferably without any coating, helps relieve CS headaches.

- Rinse the inside of your nose with normal saline (.9% Sodium Chloride dissolved in boiled or distilled water) to wash the residual smell off your nasal hairs. If it remains, you will erroneously think you are still being exposed.

- Shower as soon as possible.

- Clear the gut with Milk of Magnesia™ if the exposure was due to a food or something else that was ingested.

- Sipping hot water calms the stomach.

- If you have reactive airways disease, your physician has probably given

---

4. Prescription needed. Dr. Grace Ziem of Fredrick MD, recommends this approach. She prescribes nasal hydroxycobalamine every ten minutes, until the reaction ceases.

5. Dr. Ziem also prescribes sublingual Perque Activated B-12 Guard™ or a drop of hyddroxycobalamine under the tongue for the same purpose. At the moment there are no reports as to the effectiveness of this method. Prescription needed.

6. If you were diagnosed and treated by an environmental physician who uses this protocol, your endpoint would be ascertained and you would be supplied with the proper dose and instructions and how to administer it.

you a prescription for an Albuteral inhaler, which will open the lungs if you can tolerate it.[7]

- Regular old-fashioned tea, if you can tolerate it, also opens the lungs.

- Inhaling steam calms the lungs, which might have gotten irritated.

- Although frowned upon by most CS doctors, many people use caffeine in the form of coffee or tea to combat fatigue.

- Drink a lot of water to flush your system.

- Some people find that certain acupressure points relieve pain, or open up the lungs. A good practitioner can show you how to put pressure on them.

- Massage out muscle spasms that may have been caused by a toxin.

- Magnesium helps with muscle spasms, twitches, and restless leg.

- Some people's temperature drops when they have a reaction. Raising the temperature in a sauna or hot bath helps some break it.

- Others have reported that going into cold water, such as the ocean, during a reaction stops it.[8]

Managing a Job with CS

Many individuals with milder CS are able to work. The following are guidelines if you fall in this group.

- Do your best to obtain a relatively safe room with a window in which to work.

- Problems with cleaning materials, fellow employees or room assignment are best solved through a personal relationship with your superior.

- A few dollars to the janitor might solve a host of problems.

- As a last resort, you can claim status under the Americans for Disability Act, which requires your employer to provide you with "reasonable" accommodations.

---

7. Preservative-free Albuteral is available from Key and Abrams Royal Pharmacy

8. It is hard to understand why this works. It could be the exercise of that the shock of the cold water stimulates adrenalin or other soothing neurochemicals.

- Please note the term "reasonable."

- Perhaps you can do a portion of your job from home.

- If you are able to be up and about during the day, such as being able to work, you have been in contact with toxins that you may have masked to. Therefore, when you get back to your safe house, shower, change your clothes, sauna, eat sanely, and allow your body to detoxify so you can go out again another day.

Managing Electromagnetic Exposures

- Move away from the source, the intensity of the electromagnetic field decrease geometrically with distance.

- Take off your shoes and ground your feet in earth.

- Soak your feet in salt water.

- Soak your body in salt water. Simply add salt to your bath.

Managing Particularly Bad "Hits" That You Have Difficultly Recovering From

- Go back to basics.

- Less is more.

- As above, practice the normal drill--shower, wash your hair, sauna, Vitamin C, carbohydrates, and alkalinize your system.

- Stay in your clean room in your clean house until you feel better.

- Reduce the stress on your body by eating mono foods.

- Hydrate your system with safe water.

- Make sure that your Vitamin C levels are at the maximum as noted above.

- Some people do this by taking Vitamin C every hour until gut tolerance is reached.[9]

---

9. Many physicians do not like to stress the body this way, preferring the Perque CTM strips.

- Some people find fasting helpful. Fasting lowers the load on the detoxification system by not having to process food.

- Some people report success with various homeopathic remedies.

Emergency Kit for PWCS

The following is a suggested list of inexpensive things that everyone who has Multiple Chemical Sensitivity should have readily available. These items can help make any house safer and hopefully lessen reactions. PWCS should have a back up plan in case your safe house becomes toxic.

- Baking Soda.

- Borax.

- Barrier cloth.

- Tyvek™.

- Too Tough™.

- Aluminum foil.

- Metal tape.

- A tested safe sealer.

- A few sheets of offgassed and painted sheet rock.

- Well washed, offgassed, bedding in case you have to travel.

- Oxygen.[10]

- Charcoal mask and/or silicone respirator, if tolerated.[11]

---

10. Presciption needed.

11. Charcoal masks can be obtained from the usual sources such as Needs or the Environmental Health Foundation in Dallas. Charcoal can also be made from many different things. One may have to experiment to find the one that works best.

More Expensive, Hopefully Never Needed Items

- Offgassed tent.

- Offgassed sleeping bag.

- Sundry camping equipment.

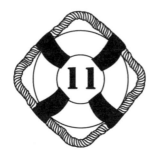

To Move or Not to Move

To move or not to move, that is the question--a question endlessly asked and ruminated about in CS community. Every chemically sensitive individual knows two things: bad air makes them sick; good air will make them feel better. Many also believe, or at least hope, that the air someplace else is better than the air they are currently breathing. When someone is having a severe reaction to chemicals, the self-preserving impulse is to run, in a desperate, frantic quest to find clean air.

The reality is that for the past twenty years, clean air no longer exists in the United States. While it is true, that some areas are better than others, all have unique local problems that cause some PWCS to get sick. The problem is that while in the midst of a reaction, one might, impulsively and frantically, climb out of the proverbial frying pan and find one's self in the fire.

Some individuals, intent on finding clean air, have spent a couple of frustrating years traveling the country, camping out or living in their car or a trailer, searching for clean air. Many ended up back at "Go" without achieving the desired results. The journey cost them money, time, and they probably got sick in one place or another that they passed through or stayed at.

Yet, if the place you live in contains known toxins in the air that are getting you sick, the only choice might be finding cleaner air. Breathing cleaner air will make most people feel better. More important is the probability that the CS will progress if the system is under constant chemical assault. The end point will be irreparable damage to vital body organs.

Moving is not an issue to blindly rush into. Much thought and research has to be done first. This chapter will give the current thinking and survey results from members of the CS community who have relocated. All have struggled with this issue. Some have achieved degrees of success, others not.[1]

The suggestions in this chapter are not meant to be a substitute for medical advice, or the advice of an environmental expert who has examined your home and environment.

To Move or Not to Move Out of Your House

- Leaving your home is the last option.

- Only move out of your house after one has ascertained that it toxic and beyond repair.

- It is best if an expert, familiar with CS, helps judge whether the house is fixable or not.[2]

- Obviously, personal finances and other resources play a large part in this decision.

- Do not leave your geographic area until you have done all you can to clean up your home.

- If you have cleaned up your home, and are still getting sicker, think about the outside air and what toxin producing industries or other such things might be in that environment and thus getting into your home.

- The progress or regress of the CS can be partially judged by the amount of chemicals accumulating in the body.

- To check on this keep a log and periodically check the chemicals, and

---

1. Consultants come and go. Some are better than others. A 2004 list can be found in Carolyn Gorman's *Less-Toxic Alternatives*, Arkansas: Optimum, 2004, p. 282. More current lists are best obtained from local support groups, CIIN, or the Environmental Health Center in Dallas, TX.

2. A list of home inspection experts and testing laboratories can be found in Gorman, p. 282.

their levels in your blood.

- It is generally believed that when recovery time from an exposure shortens, one is improving.

To Move or Not to Move to a New Geographic Location

- Only move out of your geographic area when it has been ascertained that the air contains substances that are injurious to your health.

- Inside air cannot be made appreciably cleaner than the outside air, except with an astronomically expensive filtration system. The normal commercial filters will just not do it.[3]

- If you must leave your home because it cannot be fixed, try and find a cleaner micro climate or a better, fixable home in the area that you feel most at home in.

- The psychological comfort from geographical familiarity, friends, and relatives is most helpful.

- People report that it is traumatic and difficult to leave friends, relatives, support groups, and familiar settings for the unknown.

- Many individuals who have relocated to a cleaner place end up returning back to their starting point. They become lonely and unhappy enough to trade sickness for relationship and familiarity.

- Never go from a known to an unknown.

- Do not act out of fear and panic.

- Spend time researching and talking to as many people as possible in the area that you are thinking of moving to.

- Plan how you are going to get there and where you will stay until you find a more permanent living arrangement.

---

3. Pollen and other particulates are relatively controllable with HEPA type filters. VOC's particle size is too small to be trapped by even a HEPA filter. Charcoal and Zeolite in the filtration system absorb many VOCs, but the filters fill up fairly fast. Some people are sensitive to charcoal and/ or Zeolite, and they are not as efficient as one would like. Lennox has developed a very high efficiency filter for central air systems. It is almost HEPA quality without the need for an extra powerful fan. Lennox also combines this with a titanium oxide insert that produces oxalates that remove VOCs. However, many PWCS cannot tolerate it. Try before you buy.

- Many individuals think that if they find clean air, feel better, and stay there for a couple of years, they will be healed enough to return home.

- Individuals who have tried this have found that it does not work. In the cleaner environment, they became unmasked. When feeling better, perhaps thinking they were cured, they return to their old home, they often feel worse than they felt when they were living there in the first place.

- Therefore, if you move to a new geographic location and feel better, it is possible that you will never be able to return to your old geographic area.

- Other people who moved, first felt better. Later they became sensitized to the toxins, especially the pollen producing plants, in the new area, and after a few years, had to move again.

- To reemphasize, this is a serious decision that must be carefully thought out and researched.

- Some felt better in the new location and adjusted well to the move, finding their CS improved and life was more fulfilling.

Where to Move[4]

- The place to start is to examine a 50 to 100-mile radius of where you currently live.

- Many people have found safe places in their own locale. For example if your home is on a riverbank, the air is most likely cleaner on high ground overlooking the river.

- If you plan to go further, make sure you have a plan of how to get there, and where to stay while you are looking for your final abode.

- Some people have used a trailer constructed for PWCS.[5]

- Others have lived in their automobiles.

- Safe travel guides are available from the Human Ecology Action League, but the facilities are constantly changing and there is no "safety" standard.[6]

- Green is not necessarily clean.

- Some have camped out along the way.[7]

---

4. In 2003, Robert Weinhod rated 125 U.S. cities based on quality of air, water, and ground pollution data. His top ten were: Santa Fe, NM; Rapid City, SD; Grand Junction, CO; Olympia, WA; Fort Myers, FL: Sherman, TX; Cheyenne, WY; Flagstaff, AZ; Columbia, MO; and Anchorage, AK. Weinhod ranked the states in the following order: 1. Hawaii. 2. Central and southern Oregon. 3. Coastal Oregon and the northern coastal area of California, eastern Idaho and western Nebraska. 4. Montana, Wyoming, Central and eastern Washington state. 5. Part of Colorado, New Mexico, Nevada, Utah, the Lake Superior area and the western part of Texas. 6. North and South Dakota, western Nebraska, western Kansas, and eastern Colorado. 7. Southern Florida, much of Kansas, central and eastern Oklahoma, north and west central Texas, Minnesota, Wisconsin and Iowa. 8. Louisiana, Arkansas, Mississippi, Alabama, Southern Georgia, and northern Florida. 9. New Hampshire, Illinois, most of Missouri, central Michigan, western Tennessee, central Georgia, and northwest Alabama. The eastern seacoast from South Carolina to Massachusetts and east to New York and Pennsylvania, Ohio, Indiana and South to Kentucky and eastern Tennessee were the worst. Weinhold, Robert, "Rating Guide to Environmentally Healthy Metro Areas," *Organic Style Magazine*, Sept.-Oct. 2003. However this data is several years old.

5. Advertisements for them can be found in OTT, or one can gut one and cover the walls with nontoxic material. Also see www.healthy-homes.com for reconditioned trailers.

6. http://yellowcanary.com/travelsafe/. This is only a guide as places vary in their degree of "safety" and change often.

7. Camping is free in the National Parks, and hopefully a more environmentally conscious government will ban the use of snow mobiles and quads in them.

- Camping is free in National Parks.

- The air flow in the United States is generally west to east.

- Coastal areas are favored by many except if you are very mold sensitive, as these areas tend to have high humidity, and are moldy and smelly at low tide.

- Many coastal areas, especially in the southern climates, conduct aerial spraying of pesticides on the beach.

- The west coast is not that great as it is very built up, and the western mountain range tends to "roll" back the clean air coming from the Pacific, down on the coastal land where it is then held in place by smog.

- North of San Francisco is better than south of it.

- West of the Mississippi River is better than east of it.

- East of the western mountain range is better than west of it.

- High desert works for many, except if you have breathing problems.

- Higher elevations are less toxic than lower as toxins settle down into valleys and riverbanks.

- Rural areas are better than urban ones unless you also have biological allergies to what is growing locally or if there is farming that uses pesticides.

- More open land around you is best in order to insulate you from chemical toxins emitting from neighbors, industry, or vehicular traffic.

- Land backing up to and down wind of preserved land is obviously best unless one is sensitive to the biological substances growing on the land.

- Living above the termite line is best for those who are pesticide sensitive, as homes in these cold climates do not have to be treated for termites and there is no danger of undisclosed anti-termite chemicals implanted in the walls.

- Avoid land, or houses near highways or busy streets.

- If you must be near an urban area, or some other known source of pollution, upwind of it is better than downwind.

- An urban area with lots of cement might be better for people who are extremely sensitive to flora and/or fertilizers and pesticides routinely used in agricultural areas and suburban lawns.

- Natural forests have good air, but emit tree terpenes and pollens that might bother individuals who are sensitive to them. Also, forest fires periodically break out in wooded areas, especially the Western U.S.

- Wooded areas tend to attract residents that burn the readily available, inexpensive wood for heat, thus creating wood smoke in the outside air.

- Some rural areas spray oil on dirt roads to hold the dust down.

- Some also spray herbicides on the roads for weed control.

- Avoid any area near a sewage treatment plant.[8]

- Avoid areas near electrical generating plants.

- Avoid areas near high tension wires.[9]

- Avoid areas that allow burning of garbage.

- Before committing to a new location, try and spend as much time there as possible in as many seasons and weather conditions as possible.

Obviously from the above list, there is no perfect place. All have potential problems some worse than others. As the fantasy of finding a place with perfect air to heal you dies a slow death, a difficult toxin trade off must be made. To do this, it behooves you to know what your major source of trouble is, and what the best trade for you might be. Also know that you are making a trade. There is no perfect place.

The good news is that some individuals have found microenvironments that are safe for them in places that most people regard as very toxic, even in New Jersey. This can only be done by trial, error, and local knowledge. Remember, even though other people may say that the air in an area is "pristine", or "toxic," everyone is different, and reacts to different things.

---

8. More of a problem in urban areas.

9. Unfortunately, high tension wires tend to run along the highest ground or ridge lines.

Your Home - What to Look For When Deciding to Fix it or Leave it, or Buy Another

General:

- The key to being able to create a safe house is the materials that the structure is made of and its age.

- Too old is not usually good as the wood could become moldy, and too many people have lived there leaving their toxic remains.

- Around twenty years is the optimum time for normal materials, (excluding chip board which might take much longer if ever) to have offgassed.

- New houses, even those made from the best materials, need at least six months to a year to offgass enough to be lived in, except for the very sensitive, then it needs even longer.

- If the structure of the house is good, not too old or too new, there is a good chance that it can be made safe enough to live comfortably in.[10]

- Best strategy is to have the home professionally analyzed.

- The inside walls and outside siding may look good, but who knows what is in-between.

- Send air and mold samples to a laboratory for testing.

- Have air samples taken professionally so you know what is in the house.

- Leave, or do not buy a home that has been treated for termites with one of the more toxic, never offgassing chemicals such as Dursban™ and Chlordane™. (Air samples will tell you if "toxic chemicals" are still present in the air).

- High ceilings are a plus.

- Lots of glass is a plus.

- Hard wood floors, if old enough, are a plus.

- Tile floor is a plus.

---

10. By core structure I mean, walls, floors, sheathing, insulation, siding, incoming water pipes, heating and air conditioning systems.

- Central air, preferably with more than one zone is a plus.

- Hot water baseboard heat is a plus.

- Iron hot water radiators are better than the aluminum ones generally found in houses. The fins collect dust and must be cleaned every season.

- All new radiators or baseboard heating units need a period to gas out.

- Radiant heat in the floor is the gold standard.

- Forced hot air heat is a minus and should be avoided if possible.

- If forced air must be used, make sure the system is clean, there is no possibility combustion mixture.

- Filters must be of the highest quality and changed often.

- A free standing home has a better chance of being fixed than one in a multiple dwelling such as an apartment or condominium.

- Combined living such as a condominium or apartment is possible if your unit can be thoroughly sealed off from the rest of the complex. Think watertight compartments on a ship.

- Remember that air rises in a high rise, so unless you can seal your apartment, toxins from the rest of the building will drift in.

- You should know the prevailing wind direction when picking a site.

- In multiple dwellings, the windward side unit has the best chance for success.

- So do units on the end of a building.

- In a high rise it is better to be up the prevailing wind of elevators, garbage disposals, laundry rooms, and stairwells.

- Since they are not part of the basic structure, cabinets and counters made of chipboard can be covered, or replaced with stainless steel or hardwood and thus made safe.

- Sealants and creative carpentry can make any house tighter.

- Have a HVAC expert perform a blower door test on the house for air leaks.

- If you walk into a house for possible purchase or rent and smell cooking on the stove, or fresh baked apple pie on the table, be cautious because these can be used to cover up unpleasant smells. If you see air freshener and potpourri spread around, hold your breath, walk out the door, breath in fresh air, relax and when you feel better, go on to the next.

Walls:

You should know what materials the house is made of, and how it is constructed in order to make an informed decision. The walls in an average house consist of, from the outside in: exterior siding; a vapor barrier to let the house breathe and keep water out; sheathing upon which to fasten the siding and strengthen the house; studs to nail the sheathing and interior walls to; insulation; water pipes; wiring between the studs; and an interior wall which is usually painted.

There are many houses which are made of concrete. While they can be nontoxic for most, in wet climates, or shaded areas, mold may grow. Log houses, although quaint and rustic, should be avoided. Unlike Abraham Lincoln's boyhood home, today's logs are often treated with a preservative to prevent rot, and give off numerous toxic substances. Therefore, if your house is made of logs, you might have an unfixable problem.

Exterior Walls or Siding:

- If the exterior walls are not newly painted or sided they are probably not a problem, unless made from an odoriferous wood like cedar.

- If your house is brick it will work as long as it is not shaded so the sun can keep it dry and mold free.

- Stucco is usually fine, as it is concrete, if the house is not shaded.

- Exert caution if using synthetic stucco. TEST.

- Aluminum siding is not a problem, except for people sensitive to EMF.

- Vinyl siding can work if it is old and thoroughly offgassed. New vinyl siding is very toxic.

Between the Interior and Exterior Walls:

- You must know what it is. Sometimes you can see it in an unfinished part of the house such as the attic or garage. If necessary, cut a hole in the wall and look at it. Remove a plug through the hole if necessary. It can always be replaced.

Vapor Barrier:

- Older houses, and even some new ones used tar paper, which if not old enough can be a major problem.

- Tyvek™, a relatively nontoxic vapor barrier in common use today, is usually not a problem, as it is inside the walls that are sealed with paint.

Sheathing:

- Tongue and grooved plywood is best and normal in older well-built homes.

- Chip or composite board is in common use today and the house is most likely a problem if this material has been used. These types of hard wood substitutes, almost never offgass the glues and formaldehyde they are made from.

Insulation:

- Fiberglass is commonly used and tolerated by most if old enough and the interior walls have good barrier paint on them.

- Sprayed on insulation between the walls might be tolerated by some especially if old enough, but is generally not recommended especially if new.

Studs:

- Wooden studs are fine unless you are wood sensitive.

- Metal studs are best unless you are electromagnetically sensitive.

Wiring:

- This is not usually a problem unless you have EMF sensitivities, then it is crucial.

- BX (spiral metal covering the wire) cable emits less if any EMF.

- Best would be for an expert in this field to test a house in question with a meter and make recommendations.

- Since the house is grounded, as are all the other houses in the neighborhood, there is a chance of stray electrical current wandering into your home. Again, have an expert check this with a meter.

- The major problem with wiring, in all houses, is that the wires run through very large channels from the lower level circuit box to the numerous outlets. This builder made "chimney" brings the basement air and stuff between the walls into your living space.

- The good news is that they can be sealed off at both ends.

Plumbing:

- Plastic or PVC plumbing on the supply lines are a problem.

- The plastic leaches into the incoming water.

- PVC might work for waste water, but for the very sensitive they might emit VOC's into the air.

- Older houses have copper and cast iron plumbing both of which are fine.

Interior Walls:

- Aged, painted sheet rock or wallboard works for most.

- Aged paint is usually safe except for the extremely sensitive.

- Walls can be safely painted with low VOC paint. Brands should be tested for your individual tolerance.

- Mastics used to adhere mirrors to the walls can be a problem. It would be better to use aluminum mirror channels or mirror nuts to fasten the mirror to the wall.

- Wallpaper is usually a problem. Yet, removal may cause more problems than it cures.

- However, if necessary wallpaper it can be covered with glass or foil, and therefore, not a reason to remove.

- Small troublesome areas can also be covered with glass, mirror, tile, or aluminum foil shiny side out.

Windows:

- Not usually a problem unless they leak.

- They must close tight to keep out outside toxins.

- Casement windows are best.. They are more air tight than double hung windows.

- Troublesome windows can be replaced if finances allow it.

- Window leaks can always be taped with metal tape.

Exterior Doors:

- Not a problem if the paint has aged.

- Metal doors are best.

- Exterior doors can always be replaced or altered so that they close air tight, and open out, rather than in so that on a windy day the wind forces the door closed, rather than open.

- Sliding doors, although attractive, are difficult to make air tight.

- A mud room can can be added to keep outside air from entering the house when doors open, and is valuable as a place to leave outside clothing.

Heating System:

- An electric furnace,while expensive to run, is best if you aren't EMF sensitive.

- Oil, propane or gas can be used if you can relocate the furnace outside of the house or vent it to make sure that no fumes get into the house.

- Forced air heating systems can be a problem. If you cannot afford to change the heating system to hot water baseboard, or electric baseboard, you might have to move.

- Or, don't use the central heat, use tolerated small electric heaters in the rooms you need to heat.

- Think solar and or geothermal.

Appliances:

- Gas/propane appliances should never be used for a PWCS.

- Gas/propane appliances can always be turned off at the source and replaced with electric.

Air Conditioning System:

- Very important in many climates, aside from comfort, it keeps the humidity and thus the mold count down.

- Central air with more than one zone is best, but can be made to work with one zone can work.

- The air handler should be inspected for dirt and mold and cleaned if possible.

- Air handlers tend to have fiberglass insulation in contact with the air flow. If this is the case they can be taken apart, covered, and put back together. Or a new one where the inside insulation is covered installed.

- If uncleanable, replace it or find another home to consider.

- Existing ducts need to be inspected for dirt and mold, and if found, cleaned professionally with hydrogen peroxide and new brushes.

- If new ducts are installed, add clean out ports.

- Flexduct™ is made of plastic and internally insulated with fiberglass should be avoided or replaced with TSP washed metal ducts.

- Exposed ducts can always be replaced.unlike those inside of walls.

- Vertical ducts pick up less dust and dirt than horizontal ones.

- Careful attention to filters will keep duct dust at a minimum.

- Window air conditioners tend to be made of plastic and are a source of leaks and thus problems, but again this is fixable with enough money.

- Some apartments have combination metal heating and cooling units in each room, which if clean, work well.

- If you use an evaporative cooler, make sure it is well maintained. Change the water often and dry out the pads to prevent mold growth.

Floors:

- Carpeting is not advised.[11]

- If floors are carpeted over subflooring, this can be an expensive structural problem to fix, but doable.

- For the less sensitive, old carpet can work.

- If you are sensitive to dust or dust mites, stay away from carpets or keep them well vacuumed.

- Old linoleum or old tile works for many.

- Hardwood or tile flooring or other nontoxic floor products can always be installed if the funds are available.

---

11. Some less sensitive individuals are able to tolerate so called nontoxic carpeting, and others have successfully cleaned carpets. As with everything else make sure you test any proposed carpet or cleaner.

Basements:

- Traditionally, a mold factory, which infects the rest of the home.

- It is best to select a home without a basement, such as a house on stilts or on a slab.

- Look your basement over carefully. The basement might be OK if it can be cleaned and any mold removed. Keep it dehumidified, constantly aired out, and at low pressure by using an exhaust fan. Make sure it doesn't collect water when it rains.

- If buying a house look for high water marks on the basement walls which are a sign of a past flood.

- If the walls are covered, remove a piece to look at the cinderblock. A line a few inches above the floor, hopefully not feet, will show any high water level.

Roof:

- In an older house, as long as it does not leak, the roof is usually not a problem area, especially if there is an attic between the roof and the top floor.

- Tar roofs can be a problem unless old and not in need of repair.

- One does not want to be in a house while a roof is being tarred.

- Obviously metal and tile roofs are best, but for most, fiberglass shingles work fine for most people.

- Metal roofs are noisy when it rains.

- Brand new roofing materials can be a problem until they cure.

- Best to install a new roof in the fall.

- An attic between the roof and the house is a plus.

Attic:

- If well vented, not a problem. Air tends to rise.

- An attic exhaust fan can inexpensively be installed.

- If a problem, the attic can be sealed off from the rest of the house.

Garage:

- Also a solvable problem.

- A garage in the house it is not the best, but can be made tolerable.

- The garage can be cleaned, aired, sealed from the rest of the house and the car kept outside where it belongs. It is not furniture.

- As noted in earlier chapters, it is not advisable to use the garage for storage or any item that might emit VOC's.

Area Around the Outside of the House:

- Generally not a problem unless some toxic substance has been found in the ground through soil tests.

- Bushes and trees are not good if they shade the house thus facilitating mold and algae build up, but they can, and should be removed. However, sunny is best. It keeps the house dry.

- Asphalt walks and driveways give off toxins in the heat, but if the house is well sealed, and they are old, this also might not be a major problem.

In conclusion, if the house contains large amounts of toxic materials in its basic structure, has been treated for termites, stored years of potpourri or perfume in the walls, and is moldy beyond repair, it probably cannot be made safe. If it has none of these, and is in a relatively clean air area, it probably can be made safe.

Robert S. Mayer Ph.D.

.

To Build or Buy

Whether to build a new house, or rebuild an existing house is another perennial debate in the CS community. This chapter will summarize the two views as well as dangers and pitfalls to watch out for. This chapter is not intended to be a detailed manual on how to construct a safe house, new or used, or an extensive list of safe materials to be used. Numerous, excellent books adequately cover this subject written by builders and architects of which I am not.[1] The material that follows is simply the experiences and views of the readership of OTT that responded to a request for material for this chapter. It also includes my "wish list" for what I think would be a dream environmentally safe house if cost were no object. I include it with the full recognition that many of the ideas are beyond the financial resources of the average individual suffering with Chemical Sensitivity, but offered here to shape one's thinking about how to obtain a safe house, and thus enable them to do what they can afford to do.

---

1. For example see: Bower, John, *The Healthy House*, Bloomington, IN, The Healthy House Institute, 2001 www.immuneweb.org/articles/healthyhome.html;
E-House™ (Environmental Building Consultants & Designers, 312 A Jefferson Ave, Cheltenham, Pa, 19012; Environmental Health Center- Dallas www.edcd.com; The Healthy House Institute- John & Lynn Bower, www.hhinst.com; Rousseau, David, Rea, W.J., Enwright, Jean, *Your Home, Your Health, and Well-Being*, Berkeley, California, Ten Speed Press, 1989.

General

- Choose your contractor and designer very carefully.

- Most general contractors do not understand CS. One that does is a golden find.

- If you cannot find one that understands this problem and has done it before, try to fine one that is trainable.

- Research and testimonials from other PWCS who used the architect or builder are invaluable.

- Prepare yourself. Contractors, at best are difficult. Everyone has heard horror stories even if building a non-CS house.

- Discuss and obtain agreement from them that they will respect any environmental rules you must have for your health.

- Even if you have agreement from the contractor about material and personal products they can or cannot use, the work must be monitored, as some contractors are notorious at cutting corners to the detriment of your health.

- Someone with CS should not be at a construction site. It is best for a trusted supervisor to be present during construction to prevent mistakes.

- All materials to be used, no matter what the books tell, must be individually tested by the individual who intends to live in the house.

- Whether you are pesticide sensitive, or not, care has to be taken as to where the material is purchased. Some places such as Home Depot also sell pesticides and other products that will leach into things like lumber, or everything in the store.

- Even with all these potential problems, many people have successfully built a safe new house, and many have safely retro-built an older home.

- Failures occur due to not adequately inspecting the proposed home and site, poor homework, and unfortunate choice of contractor.

Working With an Existing Home[2]

Advantages:

- If old enough, (20 years as a rough guide) the basic structure of the house had time to offgass.

- Might be less expensive to fix than to build.

- Yet, any house that has been rebuilt still needs time to offgass.

- Offgassing time for an older house is usually less than the time needed for a new house.[3]

- Utilities, roads, etc. are already in place, saving a lot of money.

- Retrofitting an existing house can usually be completed faster than building a new house.

- If you are purchasing a "CS" home, know why the individual is selling. Most PWCS do not leave safe houses, yet obviously some do.

- The best, although not always possible, chance for success in determining whether or not an existing house is safe is to find an empty one, and turn the heat up to 75 or 80 degrees Fahrenheit. This enables one to "sniff" before moving in or purchasing.

- Retrofitting can only be done if the basic structure of the house and location are acceptable.[4]

- Be wary of any house where you smell cover-ups such as fresh cooking, baking, and potpourri, or if all the windows are open when you go to inspect it.

- If the house has also been a home for dogs, cats, or birds, there are possible problems for some people with allergies.

- If there are odors from previous occupants, they must be able to be

---

2. It is best if the house can be inspected by a qualified inspector.

3. For example, even grout and tile need time to offgass. Most building material, even the safest has the manufacturing process still on it as well as what it picked up in transit, or on the supply store shelves.

4. See Chapter 11.

cleaned up or the house will not work. To help decide this, an expert can be of great benefit.

- If you are in immediate need of a place to live or want to be present while construction is going on, a temporary safe room to live in could be built next to or near the house.

- At a later time this temporary room can be incorporated into the house as a safe room, bedroom, etc.

- Some people live in a trailer, tent, or temporary structure while the work is going on.

- If you chose to do this, try to be upwind of the construction site.

- If short of funds, many toxic things can be covered with aluminum foil and metal tape without undergoing major construction.

- Be careful of "suburban housing developments." The builders often save money by using cheaper, potentially toxic things such as composite board, in areas such as inside the walls, where they are not visible.

- To look attractive, and be more saleable, developments more often than not have "perfect" lawns created and maintained with herbicides and chemical fertilizers.

- Many of these developments or communities have limiting rules on maintaining, or changing the landscaping even on your land.

- The amount of herbicide, pesticide, and fertilizer seem to be directly proportional to the price of the homes in the development or neighborhood.

- Some developments have other rules such as how often you must paint or side the outside of the house, and what materials you must use.

- The more "downscale" and/or wooded the area is, the more likely the neighbors will burn wood as fuel.

- Ample space around the house, distance from neighbors, and height are the best defenses against toxins from some other place drifting in.

- It is possible to fix up a condominium type dwelling, but it is more difficult.

- Attached dwellings often have common HVAC systems.

- Even if the system has an individual thermostat, the return may be in common.

- with any house, great care must be taken to seal off the proposed unit from the rest of the complex.

- Upwind end units probably have the best chance of success.

- Neighbors often barbeque outside in good weather.

- Neighbors often use citronella type candles or patio torches during outdoor parties.

- Although, not having any specific information, I have often thought that the top floor of a high rise, if it had a separate HVAC system, and was very well sealed from lower and adjoining units, could work.

Building a New House

- A big advantage is that you can get exactly what you need to manage your illness.

- Disadvantages are cost and time necessary to complete the process.

- Contractor, architects and designer have to be chosen with extreme care.

- Even if built with the safest of materials, new houses need time to fully offgass.

- It could take up to three years from finding a location to completed house.

- Prefabricated houses are in the news today, and are worth checking out in an attempt to save time and money but many readers report that they tried to go this route and were not successful.

- Cost escalates if attempting to build on raw land, as services and roads have to be brought in, and permits obtained.

- Therefore, it might be better might be to tear down an existing house and rebuild to use as much of the basic structure and services as possible.

- It is also possible that some of the structure might be saved.

- You could find a lot with an older mobile home on it, and have it removed, and build there, as services are already onsite.

- The end point may be worth the effort. Like most other things in this community, this is a personal/financial decision.

Location:

- The issue of location has been covered in Chapter 11. The only thing to add is that the house site should be in a place that gets good airflow.

- In choosing a site for a new house, have the soil tested to look for pesticide residue and other contaminants.

- For a new house, know the history of what the land was previously used for. Avoid land that was previously farmed or had industrial uses.

- For an existing house, note whether or not neighbors have piles of wood in their yards, or other substances that look like they burn rather than taking them to the dump. Some municipalities outlaw such burning, but sometimes residents burn them anyway.

- Obviously the best location is one that has the most open space and is located in the highest elevation in the area, or on the beach.

- Check the surrounding area carefully for sources of toxins, especially to the windward side.

General Structure:

- Unless there are very good reasons to have one, an environmentally safe house should not have a basement.[5]

- If the proposed house has a basement, it should be able to be totally

---

5. Since basements are a notorious source of mold and end up as storage for toxic items, the only reason I can see to have a basement is if you live in an area that is prone to tornadoes or hurricanes.

sealed off from the rest of the house with a separate ventilation system, and kept at negative pressure by a simple exhaust fan.

- A house built on stilts is best. Metal stilts have the added advantage of reducing or eliminating the problem of termites, ants and other crawling, climbing pests.

- Collars or guards can be placed around to stilts to keep pests out.

- Stilts allow passage of air under the house, and help prevent mold.

- If high enough, vehicles could be parked underneath, assuming a good air flow to remove any fumes from the automobiles..

- A house built on a slab is second best.

- Houses built on a slab can have a small, often unreachable crawl space underneath. You need to know how this is vented or built, and be sure it is sealed from the rest of the hours.

- If there is a crawl space, it has to be vented and mold free. Have the crawl space air periodically tested for mold.

- The garage should be separate.

- It can be connected to the house with a breezeway.

- The breezeway can also serve as a detoxifying chamber, reducing the amount of toxic material entering the house.

- The breezeway could also be use to leave contaminated clothing and other articles in.

- A one-floor ranch style house solves the problem of toxins rising from one floor to the one above it, especially if the ceilings are high and there is an attic.

- Purchase the building materials in advance as to hasten offgassing time.

- If possible, paint whatever can be painted before it is installed and store in an airy place to allow it time to offgass.

- Sources for safe materials can be found in any number of books.[6]

---

6. See: Gorman, Carolyn, and Hyde, Marie, *Less-Toxic Alternatives*, Arkansas, Optimum

- Build the garage first to store the building materials.

- If necessary build a safe room out of glass and metal to live in while the house is being constructed. The room can eventually be attached to the house with a breeze way or any other such solution.

- Another way to store the building materials is in a temporary metal frame structure similar to those used to cover boats in the wintertime.

- Like structures used to cover boats in the winter, make sure there is adequate airflow.

- Subdivide the house into airtight compartments so that if one part of the house gets contaminated, or repair work has to be done, the toxic fumes from materials and workmen can be contained.

- Each compartment should have it's own HVAC systems, so that if one area needs work, or is temporarily toxic, it can be walled off from the rest of the house.

- Metal doors and jams seal best, and they do not warp.

- All exterior doors should open out.

- The bedroom should be at the extreme windward side of the house with its own air system unless the room is downwind from toxins.

- The clothes closet must be separate from the bedroom; instead enter it from a hallway.

- The bathroom should also be separated from the sleeping and living area; enter it from a hallway to lessen the chance of contaminating the bedroom or rest of the house.

- Install exhaust fans in all closets, bathrooms, and utility room to remove toxic air outside.

- The exhaust fans must be vented outside.

- When installing exit vents, be aware of the prevailing wind.

- To prevent "blow back" install baffles on the exhausts. At very little cost, they can be set up to open when the fan is on and close when it is off.

Publishing, 2003, for a guide to resources.

- Best to have all rooms open from a hallway, rather than being able to walk through them from room to room.

- Kitchen, laundry, utility room, and guest room are best situated at the other end of the house from the bedroom, and downwind from the living area.

- Dining room and living room in the center can serve to separate the two areas.

- Offgassed, plasma computer monitors can be handled by all but the most sensitive, especially if the computer brains and printer are in a separate room.

- For little extra expense build an exercise room with a ceramic sauna.

- Build the sauna large enough so that you can lie down on the bench and sleep (without the heater on) in emergencies.

- In an emergency, the sauna so built, can serve as an additional safe room.

- You can use a futon or a number of cotton towels as a temporary mattress to sleep on in the sauna with the heat turned off.

- Build a special room, or a vented space between rooms to house electronic equipment such as computer brains, television, etc.

- TV can be viewed through a glass cut in the wall into the next room, either bedroom, living room, or both. Have speakers from the TV wired into the viewing room with you so you can hear it.

- Use a maintenance free exterior, such as glass, tile, cement or Hardy Board™, which can be obtained, pre-painted with a fifty-year guarantee, and never needs repainting.

- For the extremely sensitive, install a metal roof.

- For many, a normal fiberglass shingle roof will work as long as the layer between the shingles and roof is not tarpaper.

- In certain climates, an interesting idea is to build the roof with a large overhang to eliminate the need for gutters which need constant cleaning and eliminate freezing water backing up from clogged gutters and causing the house to leak.

- If you live in an area with a lot of snow, steeply pitched roofs would help prevent snow accumulation.

- Avoid multi-level roofs to prevent roof toxins from entering the house from windows with a roof under them.

- A full attic, well vented and sealed from the house, will prevent any odors from the roof from entering the house.

- The attic can also be used to house the air handler for the HVAC system.

- Build the house to take advantage of the environment and lessen the amount of toxic fuel you need to heat, cool and light the house.

- A glass wall, with vertical blinds, on the sunny side allows the sun to help heat the house.

- Install dark tile or marble in the opposite wall to absorb the heat.

- Put solar panels on the roof to lower the electrical cost.

- Geothermal heating and cooling system, as well as solar for electricity, will pay themselves off in about ten years and reduce fossil fuel emissions and are safer for PWCS.

- Check to see if rebates are available for solar products.

- If the house were built U shaped the center could be glassed or screened in. This can be used as a screened in insect free entertainment area.

- If the screens had glass inserts, it could be used all year around in colder climates and also be toxin free.

- The air handler should not have any exposed fiberglass insulation inside it.[7]

- Install state of the art air filtration system in the air handlers.[8]

- Use electric heat, or build a separate room, outside the house and down wind for the furnace.

- Natural gas is better than oil, because it rises up; fumes dissipate in the wind. Also there are no possible oil spills when filling the tank.

---

7. Trane™ or American Standard™ both have this option.

8. At this writing, Lennox™ has the most efficient filtration system. It is almost HEPA quality.

- Propane tanks, for heat must be located down wind of the house as propane. is heaver than air and will settle on the ground. A fan might help.

- Outside doors should open out, so wind will blow them tightly shut, rather than trying to open them in a stiff breeze.

- Construct the house so that all entrances are through a breezeway, mudroom, or vestibule to lessen the chances for toxins to enter the house.

- Install a closet or coat rack in the vestibule for outer garments and shoes.

- If possible, a changing area in the vestibule will prove very helpful.

- Also a guest bathroom and shower in the vestibule is great for obvious reasons.

- Keep this area under negative pressure with an exhaust fan to further help prevent any odors from drifting into the house.

- Install a very good exhaust fan with a shut off damper over the stove for cooking odors.

- Filter incoming water at the source for both particulate mater and chlorine.

- Use an exhaust system for all closets, bathrooms, laundry room, utility room, and kitchen; they should run 24/7.

- Keep the house under slight positive pressure with HEPA filtered intake fan to keep toxins in the wall, except when the air outside is bad, for example some one is burning.

- All rooms to have at least ten-foot ceilings for better dispersal of toxins.

- Kitchen and bathroom cabinets are best if made from hardwood or stainless steel.

- Best counters materials are: stainless steel, tile, granite, marble, or Formica covered hardwood.

Outside:

- A downwind outside patio is helpful for visitors and for cooking outside on a grill.

- Redwood is a good choice for decks and any outside wood that may be needed. It holds up well, tolerated by most, and does not have to be painted or sealed.

- Cast aluminum outdoor furniture is nontoxic.

- Do not plant foliage around the house that might shade it and thus encourage mold or mildew on or near the house.

- Cement or natural paths are better than asphalt.

- In the northeast, surround the house with an electronic fence to keep deer and other tick bearing animals away.

- In deer tick country, keep grass short; keep your self covered when walking outside.

- Inspect yourself for ticks when you come in.

- Do not worry about a lawn, whatever grows, grows, just keep it short, or let it turn to meadow if you are not allergic or worried about ticks.[9]

---

9. I have always wondered about America's fascination with these expensive to maintain, English style, perfectly manicured lawns especially since we do not play much croquet, lawn tennis, or have front lawn parties. In addition, we should not let our children play on these fertilized, herbicided, toxic areas. In my neighborhood, all the dogs do their business on my lawn since it does not have any of the above. Perhaps a reader will enlighten me.

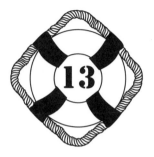

Managing CS When Out of the House

Having a safe house is wonderful, if not essential. Living in it will make you feel better and gradually improve. But unless you are totally disabled, one has to go out, shop, if for nothing else than to obtain the necessities if life. Socializing is also necessary for most humans, as well as fun, yet difficult for PWCS. This chapter will give some suggestions to help you handle visits to and from family and friends, as well as excursions out of the house and around the uninflected.

Many individuals with CS believe that exposure should be severely limited, which means staying in a safe house as much as possible, as CS is a progressive illness that has to be slowed down by limiting exposure. Other people argue that if you do this you risk falling into a black hole. Once in this "black hole," the theory is that you slip deeper and deeper until no place is clean enough. They also argue that the psychological benefits of being somewhat in the world counteract any health disadvantages. Physicians working within an immune system model believe that the immune system has to be stimulated and stretched in order for resistance to be built up.[1] Some physicians believe that you can even live in a toxic

1. Morton Teich M.D., Allergist, Immunologist, and Clinical Ecologist. Personal communication.

city, if you have a clean house.[2] Others believe that broken is broken (the detoxification system) and exposures can make one worse as exposure further damages this system and causes neurological damage. As one can see, opinions differ greatly. Unfortunately there are no studies that confirm or disprove either position. Some people benefit by living at the edge of their tolerance, others do not.

This chapter will address problems PWCS face outside of the home, while traveling, shopping, visiting friends, or entertaining visitors.

When Out of the Safe House

- Note whether you get sick from sunshine, as many PWCS do. If so stay out of it or make sure that you are covered up as much as possible.

- Lightweight sun block clothing is available from numerous sources.

- Carry your medical requirements on a bracelet or some other such device so that in case of an emergency the individuals in an emergency room or ambulance will know what to do.

- It is more self-serving to say, "I have a breathing disability" and be understood, than to explain CS during casual interactions, and be misunderstood, or perhaps judged crazy.

- It is better to use terms like Reactive Airway Disease, Asthma, latex sensitivity, and Porphyria, rather than CS if you get into trouble and have to deal with emergency health care providers or people who do not understand this illness or react adversely to any suggestion that the air they breath and products they use get you sick.

- In general large open spaces are generally better than confined ones.

- Whenever you go out, carry your own water in a recycled glass bottle, as water in glass bottles is difficult to find.[3]

- Also carry some emergency tolerable food high in carbohydrates.

- Examples are nuts, an orange, dried fruit, or some other food that is safe

---

2. Adrienne Buffaloe, M.D., and Ronald Hoffman, M.D. Personal communication.

3. Plastic bottles, especially soft ones, can leach toxins into the water.

in case your blood sugar drops.

- In a public place, sit close to an incoming fresh air source.

- Do not position yourself near a forced air heater or air conditioning vent.

- Always try to position yourself upwind from anyone using perfume or smoking.

- In a public place, if possible, position yourself as far away from other people as possible.

- If possible have a friend without fragrance on to sit next to you and act as a block from other people.

- If the place is crowded, find another.

- Pretest the air in proposed place you intend to go before you commit for a long stay.

- Many PWCS can eat in certain restaurants at off hours.

- Go into the proposed restaurant beforehand to ascertain whether the ambient air is safe enough for you.

- This also applies for most public places such as museums, etc.

- Early is usually better than late to avoid cleaning fumes and the day's toxic build up.

- In office or close settings, mornings can be worse because everyone might have freshly applied their shampoo, aftershave and deodorant.

- If you are sitting in a restaurant or some other such place and an individual with perfume walks by, do not panic, the perfume smell will most likely settle down, soon after they sit.

- If after a few minutes, it still bothers you, move to another table.

- If you want to go to meetings, classes, and/or religious services, ask if they will reserve a fragrance free area for you. As noted above, test the space first.

- If your lungs are sensitive to cold, wear a mask or cotton handkerchief over your nose and mouth when outside in cold weather to warm the air you breathe.

- If you do feel your lungs tightening, cup your hands over your mouth and nose so that you breathe in warmer air.

- If necessary, purchase a silicone (not rubber) respirator with canisters to filter out VOCs (volatile organic chemicals) when you are out of your safe environment. You might look like a bug, but health for vanity is a worthwhile trade.

- A simple cotton mask with a charcoal insert works for many people. There are many different charcoal inserts and you may have to try a few to find the one that is best for you. A note of caution, all masks reduce your oxygen intake and therefore should not be worn for a long period of time.

- If sensitive to the cotton or charcoal, silk masks with various forms of charcoal are available from the usual sources.

- When walking for whatever purpose, do so in a low traffic, and low pesticide area to reduce the amount inhaled toxins.

- Avoid: Golf courses; sprayed areas of parks and recreational areas; and beautifully landscaped lawns, and other such areas most likely to have been treated with pesticide.

- The beauty of the lawn is directly proportional to the amount of chemicals applied to it.

Traveling by Automobile [4]

- If roadside herbicide use is a problem for you, call ahead to see when the roadsides were most recently sprayed.

- When traveling, call local health departments to get the spraying schedule and locations.

- When deciding which pump to use at a gas station, check the wind direction and choose the pump positioned so the breeze will carry the fumes away from, not into, the vehicle.

---

4. This is based on having a safe vehicle as described in Chapter 8.

• Have some one else fill the gas tank so you do not have to inhale the fumes. .

• If a friend is not available, ask the service station attendant to help you. A dollar or two will help.

• If fumes start coming into the vehicle, get out and walk upwind of the gas pump.

• Keep a fold up, offgassed lawn chair in the car in case your automobile breaks down, because you might not be able to stay inside a mechanics garage.

• Keep your car windows closed and the air conditioner/heater fan set to the re-circulate position when in your vehicle to keep road fumes out.

• Avoid traveling on busy highways during rush hour.

• Drive in the car, not truck lane, on a multi-lane highway.

• Most trucks use diesel fuel the fumes of which are more toxic than gasoline vehicles.

• Whenever possible drive on less traveled roads.

• A good GPS that can find alternative routes helps you do this and not get lost.

• If necessary, while driving, wear a tolerated charcoal mask or respirator.

• Keep a portable automobile filter in the vehicle.[5]

• Keep a tank of oxygen in the vehicle. It is perfectly safe to do so, even in the trunk. Obviously, no flames while in use.

Traveling by Airplane

• First Class, if affordable, is best. Fewer people are in that area of the plane and there are only two seats per row.

• Sit next to the window an if possible have a friend who does not use fragrance sit next to you to provide a buffer space.

---

5. E.L. Foust, among others, sells portable automobile air filters. E.L. Foust Co. Inc, 1-800-353-6878, P.O. Box 105, Elmhurst, Il, 60126, www.foustco.com.

- Travel during low traffic periods when the plane is less likely to be crowded.

- Use oxygen while in the plane.[6]

- The oxygen must be supplied by the airline; you are not allowed to bring your own oxygen onboard.

- Bring your own offgassed cannula or, if necessary, Tygon ™ tubing and ceramic mask.

- If they say you must use their cannula, try it. If it doesn't work because it is new tubing, you can change to yours when they walk away.

- If needed, or as a precaution, especially in a new place, prearrange to have an oxygen company meet you with an oxygen tank at the airport when you arrive.

- Request that the individual to meet you be perfume free, and the vehicle not to have any air freshener in it.

- Prearrange to have the oxygen company set up oxygen in your hotel room as a precaution.

- When you get to your final destination, change your clothes, take a shower, and wash your hair as soon as possible.

- If you still smell the "stuff" you were exposed to, rinse your nose with salt water. Odors tend to cling to nasal hairs and make you think you are still being exposed to toxins..

- If renting a car, request one that has never been smoked in and without detailing or air freshener.

- You might have to try a number of vehicles before finding a tolerable one.

- It might be necessary to use oxygen in the rented vehicle.

---

6. You will need a doctor's prescription for oxygen, and a note that you need it on the plane. The airlines are familiar with this and will walk you through the procedure. The cost is about $100 each way.

Where to Stay

- Check the Green Lodging Directory for possibilities.[7]

- If possible, visit the proposed place of lodging first.

- Call ahead and discuss your needs to give yourself the best chances for success.

- Better chain hotels and motels usually use products with lower odors than independents.

- More and more hotels are claiming that they are "green." This might be fine, but remember, green is not clean. You must test and have an alternate plan. Many green products contain fragrance.

- Many hotels will let you see the room and test it, before you pay money.

- Carry something to cover the bed with, medical grade Tyvek™, barrier cloth, and a cotton mattress cover, all pre-washed.

- Bring your own bedding.

- Bring your own personal products.

- Carry an offgassed tent and sleeping bag for emergencies.

- These should be purchased well in advance of any proposed travel and given enough time to air out and offgass.

- It is a good idea for anyone with CS to have the above items for emergencies. Your home could bet toxic.

Visiting with Friends and Relatives

- With careful planning, and cooperative friends and relatives, a social life is possible with CS.

- One does not want to live like a hermit if possible. It is bad for the spirit.

- In advance of any visit, discuss your special needs with the individuals

---

7. *MCS Travel Directory* www.safertraveldirectory.com.

involved to ascertain whether cooperation is possible.

- Ask them not to wear fragrant products when in your presence.

- Have washed clothes available for visitors or repair people that are coming to your home, to change into if necessary.

- Keep a hair-covering device to hand out if necessary.

- In some cases, ask them to take a shower, especially after a plane trip.

- If they will not cooperate, do not waste your time trying to educate them. Not everybody is educable. Use your energy to find new friends. Obviously this is harder with relatives. This could be another Hobson's choice—your health or your relatives.

- If you are able to go to large gatherings such as weddings, plan ahead and sit between two people who have agreed to be fragrance free.

- If you want or have to go to a strange house or banquet hall, go there ahead of time to "test" the air to ascertain if you will be able to handle it.

- Often these places are not as bad as one might think; the rooms are large and usually have a good air system.

- Do not apologize to anyone about your condition; you have a disability and it is not your fault that you were poisoned.

- Don't get angry if someone forgets. It does not mean that they are trying to hurt you or don't love you. Sometimes we all forget, just move away, or if necessary, go home early.

What to Do When Accidentally Exposed Outside of the House[8]

- Do your best to stay calm. Getting angry or going into a panic will make your symptoms worse. Your job is to protect your health, not educate the uneducable public.

- If you start to get an exposure, move upwind of the source.

---

8. See Chapter 9 for more detail.

- Hold your breath or practice shallow breathing until you get into clean air.

- Find clean air.

- Meditate.

- If you have engaged in an active practice of meditation, this will be much easier.

- Listen to music, in order to change the channel in your head.

- Listen to the song in your head. If it is not there, sing to yourself.

- When you come home from shopping or some other activity where you have been exposed to something, take a shower, wash your hair, change your clothes as soon as you can in a space that is separate from your living space and until washed, leave them there.

- Pay particular attention to your hair.

- Some people find that an ionic hair blower will remove chemicals until washing is possible, and after washing help remove remaining odors.

- If you still smell something, try rinsing your nose with salt water.

- Alka-Seltzer Gold ™ will alkalinize the system and often stop a reaction.

- Hydrate yourself.

- Some people find carbohydrates help, others note that they make them sleepy. Find out what is best for you.

- Some PWCS always carry some chocolate with them. The sugar and caffeine seems to help them. Test first.

- If you get sick from a food, take a recommended dose of Milk of Magnesia™ to clear your digestive tract and reduce the transit time.

- For headache or inflammatory pain, take plain, old fashioned, non-coated aspirin.

- Use oxygen. For many people it reverses metabolic acidosis after an exposure. It replaces the depleted oxygen and prevents additional brain damage from lack of oxygen. It also assists the detoxification process.

- If you cannot tolerate the plastic cannula, age one in advance, and treasure it. To speed up the offgassing procedure, soak it in baking soda and water.

- If necessary use a ceramic facemask and Tygon™ tubing.[9]

- Exercise, or at least move. This speeds up the metabolic process, encourages sweating, and thus helps detoxify the system.

- Many people are helped by Histamine neutralization shots. [10]

- Take 1000 mg. of Vitamin C every two hours to bowel tolerance. If you do this, do not take the Milk of Magnesia™ for obvious reasons.

- Take your body temperature. Know what is normal for you. Therefore, if you are having a reaction that causes your body temperature to drop to, you can often stop the reaction by raising your temperature in a heat chamber, or hot bath.[11]

- Take a sauna to help the body eliminate the toxins.

- Remember: You have absorbed "hits" in the past and recovered. There is no reason to think this time will be different. You will recover.

---

9. Obtainable from the American Environmental Health Foundation of Dallas, 214-368-4132, www.aehf.com.

10. These have to be obtained from a physician who is well trained in treating CS. They can be self-administered.

11. This only works if you are not heat sensitive.

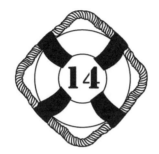

Medical Problems

Chemically sensitive individuals have a unique problem when they have a traditional medical problem. Proprietary medications from a pharmacy and prescriptions from a physician, even those that they previously used over the years, could now be contraindicated. The mainstream physician, even though he/she is bright, well-trained and well-credentialed is most likely unfamiliar with CS. Unfortunately they have not yet been trained to neither recognize nor treat the condition. More likely, they have been taught to disbelieve it, and therefore do not take the patient's claims to be sensitive seriously. They are trained and feel most comfortable when they recognize a condition they know about and thus can hand a patient a prescription with confidence that it will work.

For a PWCS, this approach could be a big error. Medicine, whether it is an over the counter drug, a prescription drug, a homeopathic formula, or a century old folk remedy very often contains substances that exacerbate CS. Obviously, there are situations where medical conditions must be treated and prescription or proprietary drugs taken. Some drugs are well tolerated by some PWCS. The problem is that an individual often does not know in advance which one medication will not cause a reaction.

The following are things that the respondents to our query have successfully used to treat common illnesses, and ailments. [1]

Basics:

- Medical problems not directly related to CS, need to be treated by a licensed physician, whether or not that physician is familiar with chemical sensitivity.

- Best chance of success is with a physician that understands Chemical Sensitivity.

- If your CS specialist is far away, CS is considered a disability; therefore, most insurance will pay for phone consultations if the doctor has seen you at least once to fulfill the legal requirement.

- If you are stuck and must see a local physician, do not try and explain CS to a physician whose mind is closed to the concept.

- Many times it is best not to even mention it unless necessary.

- This wastes time, money, and does not get you the help for which you sought out the doctor.

- Some physicians are professionally challenged and feel threatened when confronted with an ailment that does not fit into their worldview and training.

- Just find a way to work with this type of physician or find another one.

- If necessary, obtain the first appointment in the day to lessen your waiting time in a toxic office.

- Use oxygen if you must go into a toxic office.

- Ascertain in advance if the individuals examining you use fragrance.

- If they do, ask in advance if they could leave it off that day. If they won't, seek out another practitioner.

- Review Chapter 2 of this book, for more detailed general rules.

---

1. As always, the following suggestions are not a one size fits all. Everyone is different. Nor is anything in this chapter to be taken as a substitute for medical advice.

Pain:

- If tolerated, plain, cheap, non-coated, aspirin.[2]

- Aspirin is generic and can be compounded in inert filler if necessary.

- Advil™. Wash the coating off of the tablet. Swallow fast, or grind up in something you tolerate to mask the taste.

- Many PWCS tolerate morphine,for very severe pain.[3]

- Avoid the synthetic varieties that they will try and push on you and are more expensive than the original, old fashioned, yet still effective ones.

- Acupuncture—nontoxic and surprisingly effective.

- Magnesium, alternating cycles of hot and cold packs, and massage often help muscle pain.[4]

- Some people report success by rubbing Magnesium, in lotion form, onto the affected muscle.

- Elavil™ (Amitriptyline HCl) is tolerated by many in small doses for Fibromyalgia. [5]

Topical Anti-Bacterial Disinfectant:

- Avoid the high tech "sterile scrubs" as they contain chlorine derivatives.

- Wash well with soap and water, most small cuts do not need sterilization unless caused by an outdoor rusty object that might cause Tetanus.

- Apply colloidal silver on a sterile cotton ball.

- Hydrogen Peroxide.

---

2. The kind that turns to powder at the bottom of the bottle is best. Unfortunately, in this designer drug age, it is getting harder and harder to find.

3. Prescription needed.

4. IBID.

5. IBID.

- Some people can tolerate rubbing alcohol, which is germicidal.

- In general, any medication in a cream base is generally better tolerated than one in a petroleum ointment base.

- Avoid preparations containing or made from chlorine derivatives.

Oral Problems:

- For gum infections such as gingivitis, periodontists operate on the infected gums and recommend Periodex™, or some other such prescription product to keep the area clean. Unfortunately the products usually contain chlorinated ingredients and could be a problem for many PWCS, especially if used for a prolonged period of time.[6]

- Rinse your mouth several times a day with a solution of one teaspoonful of common salt in a glass of hot water.

- Better is squeaky clean preventative oral hygiene, especially flossing, to remove the tarter on which the bacteria grows.

- A water pick with a solution of hydrogen peroxide can help.[7]

- False teeth can be cleaned in Efferdent ™ or some other such product if they are thoroughly rinsed afterwards.

- An alternative is a supersonic sound cleaner, without any added cleaning fluid, available at places like Hammacher Schlemmer or other such specialty stores.

- Rinsing the mouth with non-flavored organic yogurt, and taking acidophilus can treat oral yeast or thrush.

Ear Infections:

- Swimmer's ear is common and must be treated with a topical antibiotic.

- One drop of vinegar in each ear before swimming might prevent it.

6. IBID.

7. Do not use food grade peroxide for this purpose.

- Earplugs to keep out water will also help.

- After swimming, remove any remaining water from the ear with a commercial mixture of alcohol and glycerin, if tolerated. Various brands are available at all pharmacies.

- Warm U.S.P. grade glycerin is hydroscopic and will often pull water and infections out of the outer and inner ear.

- If necessary, prescription antibiotic eardrops seem to be well tolerated.

- If you build up earwax, remove the wax periodically. Water can get under the wax and cause an infection. Some people can tolerate commercially available wax removers; others will have to go to an ear doctor and have the wax physically removed.

Eye Problems:

- A medical doctor must treat eye infections.

- Prescription medication, if needed, seems to be well tolerated.

- Avoid, unless absolutely necessary, products containing Cortisone even if the doctor informs you that they are not systemically absorbed. They are.

- Itchy eyes due to allergies can often be soothed with witch hazel, tolerated by many, applied to closed eyes on pads of sterile cotton.

- Naphcon A™ will sooth allergic eyes. It is tolerated by many, and is available without a prescription.

- Many tolerate Patanol™, for which you need a prescription.

Nose:

- Salt-water rinses can be used to rinse the nose of pollen and will lessen allergic conditions.

- Many tolerate stronger topical medication such as Afrin™.

- If a prescription nasal spray is needed for allergies, use the ones that come in hand pumps and are water based such as Rhinocort™ aqueous, although it contains cortisone and should only be used if absolutely necessary.

- For sinus infections, try inhaling steam from a facial steamer to kill the bacteria and viruses before resorting to an antibiotic.[8]

- An inexpensive treatment method is to bend over a bowl of steaming water with a towel over your head and inhale the steam.

- Irrigate the nose and sinuses with normal saline (.9% sodium chloride) in body temperature water that has been boiled first) and a bulb syringe, a neti pot, or a teapot.

- Guaifenasen, available without a prescription or compounded with inert fillers, loosens mucus in the nose, sinus, and lungs, and is well tolerated.

- Drinking hot tea, chicken soup, or water helps to get the cilia, the little hairs in these passages, beating which will help colds, and clear morning congestion.

Colds and Upper Respirator Infections:

- Only take antibiotics if the doctor is sure that it is a bacterial infection, not an untreatable virus.

- It is best, though not always possible, to have the physician culture the infection in order to obtain the correct antibiotic to effectively treat it.

- If possible take have a physician take sputum and throat cultures before starting antibiotic therapy.

- Antibiotics do not work on viruses.

- To treat a viral infection, trust your immune system, Vitamin C, fluids, rest, and tolerable medications to relieve symptoms.

- If you must take an antibiotic, resist the doctor's attempt to write for a one-dose designer drug that stays in the body for 7 to 10 days.

---

8. Conair™ makes an inexpensive facial steamer that wills offgass over time.

- If you react to it, it will take you that long to get it out of the system.

- Opt for an older drug that you have to take four times a day.

- Bactrin DS™, a sulfa drug, is tolerated by many, but for some reason not liked by physicians. It is worth a first try.[9]

- Irrigate the nose as in above.

- Steam from a facial steamer will kill viruses, as well as bacteria in the nose, throat, and lungs--try before trying an antibiotic.

- If you take an antibiotic, take acidophilus to prevent a secondary yeast infection.

- Lung medication can be inhaled with an old fashioned atomizer, or one of the newer mechanical nebulizers such as Aeroneb™,[10] rather than exposing yourself to the propellants in most commercial products.

- Albuterol is tolerated by many.[11]

- Preservative-free Albuteral for use in a mechanical nebulizer can be made up by any one of the specialized compounding pharmacies and is tolerated by many.[12]

- Zinc nasal spray and lozenges, or sucking on a zinc tablet work well to kill bacteria and viruses, if you are not sensitive to it.

- If lungs are involved, get a chest x-ray; you do not want pneumonia.

- Levaquin™ is tolerated by some.

- Cipro™ is tolerated by some.

---

9. Prescription needed.

10. IBID.

11. IBID.

12. IBID.

Pollen Allergies:

- Standard allergy shots that contain preservatives are not advised unless you have been tested for a reaction to the diluent which usually contains preservatives..

- A few allergists use preservative-free antigens and they work for some.

- Irrigate the nose frequently.

- Some antihistamines can be tolerated over a short period.

- Positive feedback has been reported for the antihistamines Allegra™ and Benedryl™.

- Generic antihistamines can be compounded with inert fillers and tested for tolerance.

- Most people get sensitive to any drug used over a long period of time.

- Aqueous based nasal sprays in a mechanical pump containing a decongestant and cortisone, even though frowned upon by CS doctors, have been used successfully by many respondents.[13]

- Neutralization shots or drops without preservatives, from an environmental doctor, work for some people.

- Some success to build up a resistance to local pollen has been reported from the use of Honey from a local beekeeper.

- Use good air filters in the house and on your air conditioner, and keep them clean. Pollen grains are large and relatively easy to filter out.

- Run the air conditioner preset to a comfortable temperature 24/7 so the air in the house is constantly being filtered.

- Do not go outside in the early morning or when lawn work is being done, and be sure that windows are closed during this time during pollen season.

- Bring in fresh air only through a HEPA filter.

- Change clothes and shower after being outside during pollen season.

---

13. IBID.

Diarrhea:

- If you are not corn sensitive, drink two teaspoons of cornstarch in a cup of warm water. It may take 2-3 cups to solve the problem.

- Eat foods that are binding such as rice, nuts, etc. Some use the "TART" diet; Toast, Applesauce, Rice and Tea.

Constipation:

- Milk of Magnesia™, the old fashioned kind, without flavoring.

- Magnesium Citrate capsules. Take upon awakening followed by a glass of warm water. Increase the dose until the desired results are obtained.

- Vitamin C every two hours until the desired results are achieved.

- A large glass of hot water and lemon juice upon awakening.

- Drink plenty of water.

- Flax seed, if tolerated.

- Old fashioned water enema.

- Many people tolerate a Fleet™ enema.

- Exercise will get the bowel moving.

- Massage the bowel area counter clockwise.

- Raising feet so you are almost in a squatting position on the toilet is more conducive to elimination and the position in which our bodies were designed for. Some call this the motorcycle position.

- If you have chronic constipation problems it might be good to take magnesium in a dose that solves the problem, every day as one of your supplements.

- Eat plenty of foods that contain fiber such as vegetables.

Acid Reflux:

- PWCS generally do not do well with the newer commercial acid inhibiting products such the Proton Pump Inhibitors, and the H2 blockers that physicians are currently recommending.

- For many, these work for a few days, and then the PWCS becomes sensitive to them.

- Raise the head of the bed.

- Take an antacid such as Alka Seltzer Gold ™ before bedtime.

- Do not lie down within three hours of eating.

- Pay close attention to your diet.

- Get a diagnosis from a CS specialist; it may be neuro-inflammation of the gut, rather than excess acid production.

- Get checked for a hiatal hernia that allows acid to move up into the esophagus and can lead to a pre cancerous condition in your esophagus.

- If you must surgically repair the hernia, it is not advised to have any foreign reinforcing mesh inserted into the body. These are made from various plastic materials and once in, cannot be removed.

Bandages:

- Curad™ band-aids are less odorous than other brands.

- Paper band-aids and paper tape do not irritate the skin as much as other brands.

- Stay away from rubberized Band-aids™.

General:[14]

- Avoid combinations of drugs, such as Tylenol™ with codeine.

- Better take a codeine tablet, and later a Tylenol™ (in either order) and see if each one can be tolerated before you take them together.

- Avoid medication that is long acting or time released, as it takes too long to get out of the system, if you have a reaction to it.

- Avoid colored or coated tablets.

- Often the coating can be washed off.

- Avoid colored liquid medications.

- Avoid prescription antidepressant medications, as the surveys show that most people get sick from them.

- Avoid liquid medications in general especially those that are colored, and flavored.

- If possible, avoid any medication that contains fillers, coloring, and chemicals whose name you cannot pronounce.

- Avoid topical medication in a petroleum base.

- Avoid steroids unless absolutely necessary, external as well as internal.

- Best is if the medication is generic and thus can be made up by a compounding pharmacy with a filler that you can tolerate.

- Medications in capsules are better than those in tablet form. They have less filers, and if clear, no coating.

- If the capsule bothers you, they can be opened and the medication mixed in water, or repacked into clear gelatin capsules.

- If your stomach cannot tolerate the capsule, talk to your doctor about the possibility of administering it rectally, nasally, or by injection.

---

14. Brand names are often used in this chapter. Many of the mentioned medications can be obtained in cheaper, generic form, and if generic, can be put into a capsule with little or no additives, and if necessary non-toxic fillers such as methyl cellulose used.

- See if the medication can be taken with a full stomach to lesson any stomach irritation.

- Check the surveys to see which pharmaceuticals have made people worse, rather than better.

- Test a drug before you take it by putting a small amount in your mouth or taking a lowered dose.

- Most PWCS do better with smaller doses of medication than recommended.

- Vaccinations are generally not recommended, however, if you need a flu or pneumonia vaccination, have the physician skin test you first, you may be able to tolerate it.

- A tetanus shot, if recommended by a physician, cannot be avoided.

- Avoid MRI, CAT scans, stress tests and other such procedures that use contrast dyes. Many can be done without contrast, even though the physicians do not like to do it this way.

- If contrast is insisted upon, skin test first. Again, the doc's hate to do this, but they will if you insist and you ask them if they are willing to take responsibility if you have a life threatening reaction. Protect your health, not the doctor.

- It is not wise to avoid routine anti-cancer procedures such as colonoscopies. Just insist on the no fragrance rule, and stay on oxygen during the procedure, and as long afterwards as necessary.

- Talk to the anesthesiologist about the anesthesia. Skin test it if necessary. Use as little as possible, depending on you pain tolerance.

- Surgical centers are generally less toxic than hospitals and easier to deal with. They have a lower risk of infection and tend to be more concerned with a successful procedure, than malpractice issues.

- Go in and smell the air and talk to the head nurse a few days before the procedure. Your major weapon is that they do not want you to have a reaction on the table and will generally accommodate you.

- If they are not responsive or respectful, find another doctor and facility. .
- Remember, they work for you, not the other way around.

Diaper Rash:

- Cornstarch if tolerated.
- Fragrance free talcum powder is obtainable from a compounding pharmacy.
- Baby wipes can be made from soft paper towels soaked in witch hazel.
- The local health food store may carry safer baby products.

Diapers:

- Washable cotton.
- Health food stores sell less toxic disposable diapers.

Sensitive Skin:

- Usually due to chemical exposure, go back to basics.
- Fatty acids taken internally are said to sooth nerve endings.
- Inhaled Hydroxycobalamine has helped some.[15]

---

15. Prescription needed.

Inflammatory Pain in the Brain:

- Aspirin. (Some have had success with Ibuprofen.)

- Klonopin™ [16]

- Neurofeedback.

- Neurontin™ has been used successfully by some, disastrously by others.[17]

- Dry heat from a sauna or a heat chamber if tolerated.

- Hot salt baths. Use sea or Epsom salt, and make sure that the water has had the chlorine and other impurities removed as they will be absorbed by the skin.

- Oxygen.[18]

Brain Fog:

- Oxygen inhaled to improve oxygen levels in the brain.[19]

- Thyroid Replacement Hormone used intranasally.[20]

Removing Odors from Your Hands:

- Rub your hands with a stainless steel soupspoon, or a piece of stainless steel while holding them under warm water.

- Make a paste of tolerated liquid soap and baking soda, scrub in.

- Use vinegar or rubbing alcohol if tolerated.

---

16. IBID.

17. Prescription needed. If you decide to try it, it would be best administered by a physician familiar with its use as there is a very specific dosage schedule and necessary lab tests for possible kidney damage.

18. Prescription needed.

19. Prescription needed.

20. IBID. This is a new therapy and very few reports have been received as to its effectiveness.

Electromagnetic Sensitization:

- Move away from the source.

- Avoid florescent lights.

- Avoid dimmer switches and rheostats.

- Use battery-operated appliances as much as possible.

- Try grounding yourself in salt water or by walking on the ground with bare feet.

- Rubber soles hold the electricity in the body.

- Turn off electricity at the source for your bedroom while you sleep.

General Ideas for Better Health:

- All relaxation techniques promote healing, such as meditation, Tai Chi, Qi Gong, Self Hypnosis, and Guided Imagery.

- Music that stimulates positive emotions has been found to be beneficial.

- Maintain a positive attitude about yourself and your life.

- Exercise helps metabolize toxins in the body.

- Walking is great, as the thigh muscle is the strongest in the body and pumps the blood throughout the system, helping to clean the toxins out.

- Eat as great a percentage of organic food as possible.

- Watch movies and read books that make you laugh.

- Keep your system hydrated.

- Get enough rest.

- Avoid stress when possible.

- Keep exposures down to the minimum.

- But, don't overprotect your immune system. It also needs "exercise."

- Stay away from designer hand cleaners, they smell, and remain a long time on the hands. Soap and water work fine, and have done so for many years.

- Carry alcohol pads, if tolerated, or a small bottle of peroxide for emergencies.

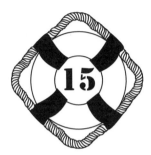

Having CS and Having Fun

Even though it may feel that way, life is not over because you were poisoned and now are chemically sensitive. Once you find ways to manage your condition, and let go of the fantasies of how your life should be, a new life will unfold. For many people the new life has been more satisfying than the old, as hard as that seems if you are at the beginning stage, stuck in your anger, or still trying to get your old life back.

This chapter will address some of the relatively nontoxic activities that can be enjoyed that will improve the quality of your new life. Obviously, each individual's degree of sensitivity will determine what he or she can and cannot do. The good news is that as one unloads the chemicals from their body, you will find that you can do more and more.[1]

---

1. The suggestions offered are general and it would be a great service to the community if you would send in any additional ideas for future revisions. Send ideas to CIIN or DRRMayer@aol.com.

Attitude Adjustment:

- This might be the most important thing that you can do for yourself. You cannot control what happens to you in life, but you can control how you react to it.

- Once the nature of the illness is accepted and the will to survive engaged, new alternatives to your old life style will emerge that will enhance and give meaning to your life. Accomplishing this will do more for you than a magic pill that only exists in fantasy.

Eating Out:

- Investigate restaurants in your neighborhood that "smell" good.

- Dine in a "safe" restaurant at off hours to lessen the chances of fragranced people sitting next to you.

- If a person with perfume walks in, you may be momentarily bothered. Very often the smell will decrease after they sit down and get settled.

- You don't have to run, or fight. You can always leave.

- Pick a table that is away from the crowd, or "smelly" people. You may need to move a few times until the best spot is found. Restaurants do not mind at off hours. If they do, find another restaurant that would like to take your money.

- If the climate is moderate, assuming clean air, outdoor restaurants are a great solution.

- Most restaurants will leave off sauces and foods you are sensitive to. They will also substitute for those that you can tolerate. If they won't, again, simply find one that will.

- Avoid restaurants that have a charcoal grill.

Food Treats:

- Buy an ice cream maker. They are relatively inexpensive and allow you to make numerous frozen deserts using milk, yogurt, or fruit juice. The resulting slushie or ice cream can be sweetened if necessary with honey.

- Freeze organic juice in an open jar. Spoon out and enjoy.

- If you are lactose sensitive, you may be able to tolerate yogurt that is made at home in a yogurt maker. This process removes all of the lactose. Homemade yogurt does not have any additives that one finds in the commercial brands, and is much less expensive.

- If you are allergic to milk, you may be OK with goat or sheep products.

- Whipped cream can be made at home without additives and preservatives with a whipped cream machine and a CO_2 cartridge.

- Soda can be made with pure water in a soda siphon. It can be simple seltzer or flavored with anything you can think of that is tolerated, such as fruit juice.

- You can purchase yeast free bread.

- You can make organic yeast free bread with a bread machine.[2]

- Freeze small portions of cooked preservative-free bacon, pork, or turkey. Take out with you in a cooler if you get hungry while out of the house.

- Freeze bananas, or grapes, or any fruit for a frozen, sweet snack.

- Buy and freeze these fruits in season for the best taste and later use.

- Nuts, cheese, and fruit are easily transported, especially in an insulated bag.

- Buy a waffle maker, and make creative mixes for allergy free waffles, like plain buckwheat flour and water. Top with honey or maple syrup.

---

2. Breadmasters, 562-695-3443

Friends:

- Try to think of things your friends like to do, that you may be able to try to do with them, especially outdoor activities.

- If you join others at an event, take your own transportation in case you have to leave.

- Find out about outdoor concerts, art shows and sporting events.

- It is obviously best to do what ever you can to maintain a social/family network. This is often a problem as individuals who are not chemically sensitive, or in denial, use products, which might make you sick, and either, do not understand the problem or will not cooperate.

- Cooperation is better than understanding if a choice has to be made.

- Do not waste energy trying to reason with the unreasonable, convert the unconvertible, or educate the uneducable.

- In the immortal words of Simon and Garfunkel, "People hear what they want to hear and disregard the rest."

- If friends and relatives refuse to follow basic rules when visiting or entertaining you, find new friends.

- Supply guests with a fragrance free product kit, which you can make up containing such items as shampoo, sunscreen, deodorant, moisturizer, and laundry detergent.

- If the weather is good and the ambient air clean, it is often better to visit with friends outside, on your, lawn, deck or in a predetermined safe public place.

- Keep a supply of "safe" sun block in the house for needed occasions.

- If the product is not completely safe and the guests must use it, stay upwind of them.

- Keep a supply of Tyvek ™ suits such as surgeons or mechanics use, or cotton sweat suits in the house so that workman and guests can put them over their clothes, which have probably been washed with non-tolerable products.

- Have guests shower with your soap and change into safe clothes that you have previously washed in your detergent.

Gardening:

- Gardening is great for obtaining fresh air, exercise, and is a life affirming project.

- Gardens make the home look pretty.

- You can grow your own organic vegetables and herbs.

- For indoor gardening, try hydroponic gardening, no dirt, and no bugs. You can grow spices, tomatoes, salad greens, flowers, etc.[3]

- Indulge your creativity with different types of plants, rocks, glass spheres, solar lights, etc.

Ideas to Control Pests and Weeds:[4]

- Ants: Grow mint or bay leaves, if you can tolerate the smell, around the outside of the house.

- Place containers of boric acid, sugar, and water around. The ants eat the sugar and take the poisonous boric acid back to the nest where they will be cleaned by the other ants. Soon they will all die.

- Ants will not cross a cinnamon line.

- Cornmeal kills regular ants. They eat it, and drink water, since they can't emit gas, they swell and then die.

- Dishwashing soap kills ants and stops them from coming in; it also kills fleas and ticks and deters scorpions from coming in through the doorway if squirted on either side of the door jam and under the doorway.

3. AeroGarden ™ is a self-contained idiot-proof system that will work anyplace, even in a closed closet. There are many others, check the web or your local yellow pages for a specialty hydroponic garden shop. At least you know pesticides will not be needed. http://www.officialaerogarden.com/default.aspx?adid=ggl1002.1

4. See the website: www.beyondpesticides.org, and www.pestsicide.org.

- Relatively nontoxic ant killers are available.[5] As always, test.

- Human urine will repel smaller animals than you.

- Purchase electronic or battery operated bug repellants at almost any hardware or warehouse store. They work great if you are not EMF sensitive. They also work against other rodents.

- Seal all containers and entry points into the house.

- A mixture of diatomaceous earth sprinkled around gardens works well for pest control. It is made from smashed microscopic sea organisms that have sharp edges and slash bug bodies and snails.

- Old fashioned flypaper.

- Use a vacuum cleaner hose to suck up bugs on the walls even while they are flying.

- Purchase a cordless rechargeable hand-held vacuum for the same purpose.

- Set wide mouth jars with wine and a tablespoon of honey and water around. Bugs will enter and drown.

- Warm soapy water thrown on wasps, hornets or their nests will kill them before they can take to the air.

- A yellow light will keep mosquitoes and other small flying insects away.

- A steamer will kill the weeds in cracks in cement walks.

- Safe spray to kill weeds: mix a gallon of white vinegar with a cup of sea salt in a weed sprayer. Avoid spraying plants you want.

- If you must use a pesticide company-use a reputable organic pesticide company that uses integrated pest management.

- If they want to apply a product, make sure to check it out for yourself.

- For termites, use boric acid gels and diatomaceous earth.

- Oil of cloves around your house helps repel insects if you can handle the smell.

---

5. Peaceful Valley Farm Supply, 888-784-1722.

- Beer in bowls will attract wasps and either they drown or the alcohol will pleasantly kill them.

- The best weed killer is you. Pull them up. The advantages are a better garden and a healthier body.

Reading:

- New or used books can be made tolerable by allowing them time to offgas.

- One can read toxic books using a reading box, or with a piece of cellophane or glass over the page.

- Reading toxic materials is doable outside.

- Well outgassed out fragrance free magazines.

- Books on tape or CD.

- Books for the blind will allow you to rent from their library if you get a note from a doctor stating that you are disabled.

- You can download almost any newspaper to your computer, handheld device or some of the new cell phones.

- Many books and newspapers can be downloaded to a reading tablet, such as Kindle or iPad for a fee.

Computer:

- A computer is of great benefit, if you can find a way to tolerate one, as discussed earlier.

- With a computer you can play games, join chat rooms, and make contact with innumerable people as well as obtain information that you would have previously had to go to the library for.

- Many people are sensitive to non-ionizing electromagnetic radiation emitted by computers as well as the plastic cases, especially when new.[6]

---

6. Monorail Model 7245 Personal Computer™ has a liquid crystal display which emits virtually

Watching TV:

- If you have trouble watching TV, try an older well-used set.

- If this does not work, put the TV in a box with a glass front and the small speaker removed from the set and led outside. If the TV has audio outs, you can connect them to a stereo, and have only the speakers in the room with you. If the TV has a headphone jack, a computer speaker, or one of the new lightweight, small, hard plastic head phones will work.

- Vent the fumes from the TV directly outside with a small fan.

Hobbies and Nontoxic Things You Can Do:

- Study nature and observe the wildlife near you, such as butterflies.

- Knitting, use cotton, bamboo, silk or cashmere yarn if you are sensitive to wool.

- Jewelry making, by knotting or stringing glass or crystal beads as well as pearls. Also, wire design with a round nose plier and wire cutter can create some great pieces. Supplies can be attained from any art and craft supply store or online.

- Picture puzzles.

- Computer games.

- Play games online with online opponents.

- Sewing your own clothes, gifts or household items.

- Sewing wall hangings or quilts.

- Sculpting out of stone with a mask.

- Clay sculpting. Wear nontoxic gloves.

- Start a telephone support group.

- Woodworking, if wood does not bother you.

---

no radiation and no smell from outgassed models. Apple computer has a solar power pack for its Powerbook™ Allermed has stainless steel computer cabinets, and The Safe Reading and Computer Box Co. has galvanized steel computer and TV enclosures.

- Painting or drawing with nontoxic materials.

- Make a collage with materials that do not bother you.

- Wire sculpture.

- Carve soap sculptures.

- Visit a craft store and get additional ideas.

- Cook or bake creatively. A side benefit is that you will eat healthier and cheaper.

- Digital photography.

- Learn computer art, design, graphics, and website design.

- Bird watching and feeding.

- Look for classes online, on the computer or on tape or DVD.

- Yoga or other health oriented classes.[7]

- Fishing.

- Listening to music.

- Learn to play an instrument.

- Creative writing, poetry, short stories, and/or biographical.

- Research your family tree.

- Look up old friends from earlier in your life or other locations you lived.

- Write to a pen pal or two, online or snail mail.

- Study the history of where you were born or live.

- Start collecting an item you enjoy, such as glass hummingbirds.

- Find others who like to walk or bike.

- Learn about any volunteer activities you may be able to do, some involve going to their location, others can be done from home.

---

7. Notice of yoga and other classes can usually be found posted in health food stores. Some of these may be health conscious and already using nontoxic cleaners.

Getting involved in a good cause might help with feeling isolated and unproductive.

- Try online dating if you are single.

Pets:

- Own one if you do not have an allergy to dogs, cats, or birds, obviously they have proven to be great companions for thousands of years.

- If allergic to the above, try a rabbit, I am told they make great companions.

- There are dogs that for some are hypoallergenic, as they do not shed, such as poodles.

- If you cannot own your own, make friends with a neighbor's dog.

- Feed a stray cat that lives outside. Keep it a little hungry and it will clear your property of mice, rats, and small rodents.

- If you need an inexpensive small pet, try a goldfish in a bowl, colorful and some company. An additional benefit is that watching fish swim in a bowl or tank is a very relaxing activity.

Exercise:

- Exercise is fun and can help the body remove toxins.

- Simple hand weights are adequate.

- Get an exercise bike for bad weather days.

- Put on some music and dance, move, march in place. This will burn toxins and calories as well as make you feel energized.

- Used, offgassed equipment might be best if it does not have any perfume or other smells from the past owner that cannot be cleaned off.

- Walking in a nontoxic area is good exercise and a pleasant experience.

- Avoid golf courses and other recreation areas where pesticides may have been sprayed.

- Swimming in salt water is excellent exercise, nontoxic, and a good way to get rid of toxins and absorb minerals.

- If you are near a beach, it is a great place to walk, as the air is usually clean and filled with minerals that will be absorbed through your skin.

Travel:

- Travel is possible even though you have CS.

- You can take day trips to interesting locations nearby.

- You can travel by car to relatively safe hotels.[8]

- It might be possible to retrofit a travel vehicle or purchase a used one.

- Do not purchase any travel vehicle until you have self tested it to see if it is safe for you.

- You might find a tent you can tolerate and be able to go camping.

---

8. See the safe travel directory, www.safertraveldirectory.com

Appendix

Treatment Efficacy In Multiple Chemical Sensitivity[1]

The Highest Rated of 101 Treatments—Rank by % Helped

Treatment	%Harmed	%No Effect	%Helped
Chemical-free living space	.6	4.5	94.8
Chemical Avoidance	.8	4.7	94.5
Relocation	7.4	6.0	86.6
Air Filter	6.0	11.8	82.
Oxygen for exposure	7.3	14.2	78.4
Charcoal Mask	12.8	9.8	77.4
Support Group	8.7	15.5	75.9
Aluminum Foil to seal off gassing	7.6	14.7	74.4
Rotation Diet	5.7	22.1	72.2
Oxygen Therapy	10.7	20.3	69.0
Acupressure	4.5	28.3	67.2
Prayer	1.4	34.4	64.2

---

1. Abbreviated from: Gibson, Pamela, Elms, Amy, & Rudling, Lisa, "Treatment Efficacy in Multiple Chemical Sensitivity; Self-Reported Treatment Efficacy in 917 Persons with Multiple Chemical Sensitivity," Paper present at the Chemical Injury Information Network 2001, MCS Conference, Santa Fe, New Mexico, August 13-15,2001.

Psychotherapy to cope with MCS	4.5	24.1	65.0
Herbal Medicine	11.8	25.5	63.8
Massage	8.7	32.5	58.8
Craniosacral work	6.6	36.6	56.7
Reflexology	4.8	38.5	56.6
Touch for Health	3.8	41.8	54.4
Nambudripad desensitization (NAET)	7.6	38.6	53.9
Acupuncture	10.2	36.0	53.8
Meditation	2.8	43.3	53.8
Magnesium Supplements	6.1	41.4	53.4
Acidophilus	4.1	44.0	52.0
Other Vitamin C	9.5	38.8	51.7
Chiropractic w/applied Kinesiology	6.8	41.7	51.4
Qi Gong	9.8	40.7	49.6
Yoga Asans (postures)	8.9	41.9	49.3
Other mineral supplements	7.7	43.4	48.9
Milk thistle seed	9.7	41.6	48.7
Reiki	7.5	44.6	47.8
Polarity Balancing	8.2	45.9	45.9
Traditional Chiropractic	8.3	47.4	44.3
Faith Healing	4.7	51.6	43.8
Vitamin E supplements	7.2	53.1	39.6

About the Author

Robert Mayer, Ph.D.

Dr. Robert Mayer was born in 1934 in Newark, New Jersey. After receiving his undergraduate degree in Pharmacy from Rutgers University in 1956, he practiced pharmacy. During his years as a business owner, he owned two drug stores, and a number of dry cleaning stores. He believes the highly toxic chemicals used in the dry cleaning industry caused him to develop Chemical Sensitivity (CS). In 1962 he, sold his businesses and entered graduate school at Rutgers University, receiving a PhD in History in 1967.

In 1976 he obtained a post doctoral degree in Psychoanalysis and Psychotherapy from the American Institute of Psychoanalysis and Psychotherapy, thus becoming a Psychohistorian and a clinician. During these years he was a tenured Professor of Psychohistory at Kean University, Union, New Jersey, a fellow, senior instructor, and Director of the clinic at the American Institute, as well as in private practice in New York City.

Dr. Mayer's private practice specialized in dissociated states, Multiple Personality Disorder, and Post Traumatic Stress Disorder (PTSD).
He was a pioneer in the treatment of dissociated states and childhood sexual abuse, and considered one of the experts in New York. He was interviewed on national television over 123 times by such prominent interviewers as Mike Wallace on 60 minutes, Larry King, Phil Donahue, Sally Jesse Raphael and others.

In addition, he has written over seven books including *Through Divided Minds*, Doubleday, 1988, and *Satan's Children*, Putnam, 1990. He has also written numerous articles for *Our Toxic Times*, and for the *Human*

Ecology Action League (HEAL) on various subjects related to MCS (reffered to as CS in this book).

Dr. Mayer realized that he had become chemically sensitive in the 1980's, consulted with and was treated by every physician in the New York Metropolitan area that supposedly had expertise in this illness without success, or receiving a definitive diagnosis. In 1991, he was finally diagnosed by William Rea M.D., and spent six weeks at his clinic in Dallas, Texas.

At one point his illness became so severe that, after trying to make four different New York City dwellings "safe," he gave up on the city and moved to the New Jersey shore. There he reconstructed a "safe" house on the beach, and recovered enough to resume teaching at Kean and his practice in New York.

At present he has retired from his practice in New York, but still teaches at Kean University. From his own life experience with CS and professional training, he is well equipped to help those with CS adjust to and learn to survive and thrive with CS. His current practice consists of phone consultations or in-person sessions restricted to those with chemical sensitivity.

About the Editor

Treesha deFrance

Born in Brooklyn NY, Treesha deFrance graduated from Millersville University in PA, summa cum laude, with a BA in psychology in 1987. She has a certificate in Gestalt Psychotherapy and Pastoral Care. At age 38, while studying art, she acquired CS, which she believes was brought on by the toxic art chemicals. After 2 years of seeking medical help, she was diagnosed with CS. She made numerous lifestyle changes, including moving to safer housing and practicing avoidance, and began to have better health.

Since acquiring CS, many of her efforts have focused on helping others with CS. She founded the Lancaster Area Chemical Injury/Sensitivity Support Group and was its leader for 8 years. Ms. deFrance edited the Philadelphia PA HEAL chapter newsletter, "CEASE", in the late 90s. She has volunteered for 3 CS related non-profits, The Dispossessed Outreach Project and the Prescott Valley AZ New Horizons Independent Living Center. Ms. deFrance writes the monthly Research Profiles in "Our Toxic Times" for the Chemical Injury Information Network.

Ms. deFrance helped incorporate Dewey-Humboldt, AZ, and was its first appointed, then elected councilwoman. As the Chair of the Town's Environmental Issues Advisory Committee, she continues to work for public health, clean air and water there.

Post-CS, artistically, she is a member of the Creative Canaries, an international network of artists with MCS, www.creativecanaries.org. In addition to her MCS comic books (www.myspace.com/mcscomics), she has illustrated 2 books, *PA Wildlife Limericks* and a Dutch book on MCS, *Als Chemische Stoffen en Geuren je Ziek Maken*. She has had her poetry published many times and has had her artwork and jewelry and photography in shows. An avid musician and music producer at her home studio, Ms. deFrance recently produced her first CD, *Kaleidoscope, An Anthology of Women's Music*, an all-female, all-original collection, for which she also did the art. Her ongoing musical productions can be found at www.myspace.com/treeshasmusic, including some songs about life with CS.

She currently lives in the beautiful high desert of Arizona, far from her 2 beloved sons and where she hoped life would take her. She enjoys better health there and pursues her many interests, although after 20 years, her CS is still with her.

About the Designer:
Randy Mayer

Randy Mayer is an accomplished, award winning artist, illustrator, sculptor, jewelry maker, graphic designer and environmental consultant. She graduated from the Fashion Institute of Technology in 1973, spent a number of years as an illustrator, and designer, and later became a professor there.

She contributed many of the ideas for this book, which came from her experience helping to heal her CS, afflicted husband. She also helped edit this book, as well as designed and produced the overall layout, format, and the cover.

She is currently engaged in illustrating, for books and magazines as well as freelance designing. Randy is also in the process of writing and illustrating her own book. Her work and bio can be found on her websites; illustrationation.com, randymayer.com, and randyleedesigns.com.

Randy can be reached at randy@randymayer.com.

Notes: